THE STUFF YOURSELF DIET

By

FREDRIC NEUMAN M.D.
And WARREN GOODMAN

Introduction

A lot of diet books have already been written— by my count, thirty-seven thousand, six hundred and two. (And I may have missed one or two.) Therefore, I cannot claim that what the world needs right now is still one more diet book, especially when it seems that all the others were unsuccessful, at least measured by the standard of helping people lose weight and then remain at their proper weight. Why bother to write still one more?

I write this book precisely because the other books were unsuccessful. The rate of obesity, and, therefore, diabetes, is rising very quickly and caus-ing very serious medical problems and very real suffering. When excessive weight is extreme, it can cause both psychological and physical disability. Besides physical illness and emotional distress, there is a financial cost to obesity. According to a report I read yesterday it is over a trillion dollars a year. (How do they figure this stuff out?) And there are a lot of people in the world who may not be technically obese but who consider themselves "overweight"(fat.) There is a real need for developing a workable program to help people control their weight. I have some reason to think that the methods described in this book work. Of course, all those other diet books were written by people who presumably had the same hopes, and they turned out to be wrong. Actually, maybe not all of them did expect to succeed. After all, some diets were exactly the same as others that had gone before, but had a new name, usually something catchy, like "The Scarsdale Diet." (Is Scarsdale famous for having skinny residents?) Certainly, the approach of each new book was similar to that of the previous ones. It is time now for something different.

Dieting is interesting because it is an example of how people have an extraordinary amount of trouble changing the way they live. I am not talking just about dieters, or about someone who is addicted to drugs or nicotine, for example, but to *anyone* who for some reason or another wants to change, or, perhaps more accurately, *should* want to change. This is the central problem of every kind of psychotherapy— and addressing it is the central purpose of psychotherapy. People say they want to get somewhere, *and yet they will not do those obvious things they need to do to get there!* Scolding does not help. We all resist change. We all act on occasion perversely against our best interests. Everyone is guilty of doing this sort of thing in one circumstance or another. This book describes some of the strategies that are used in the context of therapy, but, really, in many other situations also, to help overcome this stubbornness of habit.

I would like at this point to offer some reasons why the reader might find my ideas about dieting credible. I have been a psychiatrist for over fifty years. During the course of that time, I have had to counsel hundreds of people who were dieting, thinking of dieting, despairing of dieting and some who were actually dieting successfully. In addition, I designed an obesity clinic many years ago for a medical school. I have also over the years had to treat bulimia and anorexia nervosa, two interesting and potentially very serious illnesses that arise in the context of dieting. In short, I have had considerable experience helping people to control their weight. I make a point of my professional experience because I have not had the sort of experience some people value: that is, I have never been fat. In particular, I have never been 150 pounds overweight and lost it by finding the exactly right formula. I take no credit for being at my proper weight throughout my life. The fact is, I don't really like to eat. The reader must decide whether my never having been fat undermines my understanding of how it feels to be fat and what to do about it.

For those of you who do feel uncertain of my opinions about weight loss for this reason, I have good news. My collaborator, (who is also my son-in-law) is fat, or used to be fat, anyway. He knows what it is like to diet. He loves food. I don't know how he married into our family. When we talk about places we have been to or plan to visit, he talks about restaurants. And *he* is the guy who has designed all the recipes in these pages.

The main point of this book is simple. The failure to diet successfully, is a *psychological* failure and does not depend on the nutritional details of a diet. In order to succeed, psychological interventions are required.

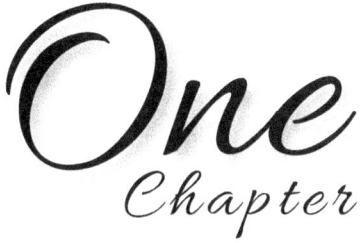

Chapter One

hen I say psychological interventions are critical to achieving weight control, I do not mean to imply that I think obesity is psychologically caused. There are many causes, many of which overlap and most of which are not well understood. Probably, there are some people who do overeat for purely psychological reasons. Certainly, there are some who claim that they eat only when they are under stress, or when they are frustrated, or when they are bored. And, of course, dieting always occurs in a psychological context since people who are overweight usually feel guilty about eating too much or the wrong things; and, often, they feel ashamed of their appearance. Their state of mind is always relevant even if their excessive weight has other causes. There are a few, I think very few, whose behavior suggests that they want to be unattractive since being overweight protects them from having to deal with certain situations that might for one reason or another make them feel uncomfortable, for instance, the prospect of a sexual encounter. Explanations of this sort are given too readily by therapists, though. The same sort of explanation may be given to explain away any kind of emotional problem, i.e.,"He wants to be rejected. That's why he behaves that way." It is one more way to blame patients for whatever problems they have. If it is their fault, we don't have to feel so bad about their feeling bad.

It is easy, also, to blame the parents of an obese person by claiming they taught their child bad eating habits. They may have encouraged their children to eat everything on their plate. Or they may have rewarded them with food, usually foods like ice cream or cookies. These are foods that are thought by others to be inherently bad. Indeed, some people do reward themselves in later life with food when they have been successful in some way, even, perversely, if that success is having been able to diet successfully for a period of time. If there are some people who seem to eat purely for psychological reasons, they are relatively few compared to those who eat, they say, simply because they are hungry.

PROPER WEIGHT

How much should someone weigh? This question is tied up with another question: why should someone want to be at his or her proper weight? There are two reasons:

One: Being overweight is regarded by most people as being unattractive, just how unattractive depending on just how overweight someone is.

Two: Being overweight, and being very overweight, in particular, causes serious health problems. This risk to health is widely recognized, but is much more serious than most people think.

For every person who diets for health reasons, there must be ten who diet because they want to look better.

THE RIGHT WEIGHT TO BE ATTRACTIVE

The desire to be attractive is natural enough, in fact it is universal. Animals all the way up and down the animal kingdom invest a tremendous amount of effort making themselves attractive: putting colored substances on themselves and preening and so on. Physical extremes of one sort or another are not attractive. Too short, too fat— and too skinny, for that matter— are not attractive. But, clearly, there is a fashion in such matters. The fat ladies in a Ruben's painting were painted fat because that was thought to be attractive. Prehistoric figurines of women were portrayed fat, even very fat. Similarly, fashion models who are surely too thin to be attractive to some men are surely attractive to others—and appear attractive to women also; otherwise no one would hire them to be fashion models. But let's talk about too fat. No one who is otherwise healthy goes on a diet to gain weight. Except, of course, body builders—which proves that I am wrong. Some people do find particular extremes, muscles, I suppose, or really big breasts, to be attractive. Now that I stop to think about it, I know of a club of 400 pound women who get men calling up for blind dates. There are not many such men, however.

Some facts:

1. There are a number of married men who have complained to me that their wives are too embarrassed by their weight to have sexual intercourse with a light on. They go on to say to me (why would they lie to me?) that they find their wives very attractive. So, we may conclude by this that many women have an exaggerated concern about how their being fat affects men and, in particular, their attractiveness to men. I might say in this connection that if a seduction has gotten to the point where a woman has taken off all her clothes, it is not likely that a man is going to be deterred by *any* physical impairment she may have.

2. There are women who are so discouraged by their appearance that they make no attempt at grooming or makeup. They become unattractive, not because they are fat, but because they make no attempt to be attractive. Not infrequently, they snarl at men in the bargain since they are angry at being rejected, even before they are rejected.

3. Over the years, I have noticed that women commonly come to a therapy session and apologize for looking fat and unappealing and at other times tell me that they know that the three pounds they lost last Friday make a difference. Today they look good, they tell me. Usually, I can't tell the good days from the bad days. I think I should be able to tell, because on the good days, they dress more carefully; and they are smiling at me, which I think should make them more attractive. But the fact is, I can't tell. The differences that seem obvious to them are too subtle for ordinary human beings

to take note of. I warn people who are dieting that their weight loss usually goes unnoticed until they have lost about one eighth of their body weight.

4. By my reckoning, about 5% of men and women are so good-looking that pretty much everyone finds them attractive. These are people who get noticed when they walk down the street. Another 15% of the population are *really* unattractive. This group is interesting to me. Many of them are not ugly because they are disfigured in some way. They seem to work at becoming ugly. They may be unkempt, poorly-groomed, slack in posture, and slovenly in dress and manner. Some whine unpleasantly. Perhaps some of these people feel bad about being unattractive, but most of them, as far as I can tell, do not care. If they did care, I suspect they might not be in this group.

That leaves everyone else. *Everyone* in the middle 80% of the population will discover the same thing: some people will find them attractive, and some people won't. Fat or skinny, long hair or short, wearing glasses or contact lenses, or fake eyelashes, or designer sunglasses—it doesn't matter. Some people will find a particular person attractive and others won't. Everyone has to adjust to this fact.

By the way, I have spoken to those few who are beautiful or handsome and asked them what it was like to be especially attractive. They say it only helps in the first few minutes when they meet someone. Maybe they are not entirely aware of the effect of their appearance. It is well-recognized that attractive people get paid more at work, for instance, than others; but, even so, their lives are not dramatically different from everyone else's.

The bottom line: Except for people who are very fat—so fat that that is the first thing anyone notices about them—how fat or thin someone is is not likely to impact his or her physical attractiveness in any significant or predictable way. Therefore, the proper weight for someone who is trying to look his or her best is within a range. Most people do not recognize that their appearance does not change noticeably—noticeable to other people—if they gain five, or even ten, pounds.

Some people say they want to be at their proper weight, usually thin, not because they are anxious to attract someone else, but for its own sake. They want to look good just to please themselves. I was inclined, when I first heard someone say this, to dismiss it out of hand. I tried imagining that particular woman stranded all alone on a desert island, brushing her hair 200 times in the morning, as she usually did, putting on makeup, and squeezing into her favorite bathing suit, just to please herself; and I couldn't do it. I realize now that she wasn't trying to fool me or herself; the idea of being an attractive person can become so much a part of oneself that being true to oneself *means* being as attractive as possible.

Take the matter of plastic surgery. A patient, usually a woman, confides in me that she is planning on having plastic surgery. Usually, I can't guess before she tells me exactly what part of her body she wants to fix. I may think she is unhappy with her nose—although it looks fine to me—but it turns out she wants to get rid of some fat covering her thighs. I have had this said to me by a *beauty contest winner.* In my experience, most people who do have plastic surgery are pleased by the result *even though they recognize that no one else notices the change in their appearance.* So it is true that people, at least some people, want to look just right in order to please themselves. But they should know that when they struggle to reach the exactly right weight, they are trying to score a bull's-eye on a target no one else can see.

THE RIGHT WEIGHT (OPTIMUM WEIGHT) TO BE HEALTHY

There are scales readily available which give a range of "proper" weights for height and sex, and age. These are based on averages; and they may not reflect the most desirable weight for an individual, if for no other reason that there are variations of other physical parameters in each person which may affect the ideal weight. Other physical measures are also commonly presented as having a "normal" range. Usually, "normal" is taken arbitrarily to include the middle 90% of a particular group, meaning that the top 5% and the bottom 5% are "out of the normal range."

Patients are often distressed to discover that one laboratory result or another is out of the normal range; and it is difficult sometimes for their doctors to reassure them that such a result does not mean that they are sick. For that matter, having a physiological measure that is within the normal range does not mean that that level of whatever is being measured is healthful.

For example, for years I was told that my cholesterol level of 260 mgm/dL was normal simply because it was not in the worst (highest) 5%. It turns out that the lower the cholesterol level is (even within the normal range) the less likely is someone to develop heart disease. For every one percent total cholesterol is lowered, the chance of a heart attack goes down by 2%. My cholesterol level was high enough to cause coronary artery disease even though I had no other risk factors for that condition.

At the same time, my bilirubin test was always very elevated. This has no clinical significance, and I was never sick as the result of it.

In short, being in, or somewhat outside of, the normal weight range does not mean someone is at their optimum weight. Deciding what that weight is, however, is controversial. I don't recommend a lot of time spent figuring out someone's Body Mass Index (BMI} This is a figure that measures height against weight. It seems to me like measuring the distance to the moon in inches.

CALORIC RESTRICTION.

For many years now it has been known that many animals, ranging from simple organisms like yeast all the way up to mammals, can extend their life span, even their *normal* life span, by restricting their caloric intake. Mice, for example, given less than their usual caloric intake, live longer, and *healthier,* than mice from the same litter that have eaten a more typical diet. Their lower caloric diet must be supplemented, however, by vitamins and other nutrients they might not otherwise get from their diminished diet. At a time when most mice are enfeebled from old age, and moribund, these mice are healthy and sexually active. If caloric restriction is started at birth, typically it produces a small animal; but it produces no other obvious bad effects. If the diet is started after physical maturity, there is no effect on size, although the ability to reproduce is diminished. In fact, this response to caloric restriction has developed through evolution as a way of dealing with famine. There is no point reproducing if there is not enough food to sustain the next generation. It is as if the animal has decided to live longer to wait for the famine to be over.

The general consensus is that caloric restriction is too difficult to be successful in human beings. People are hungry all the time. Nevertheless, there are some who do stick to this diet. They are often researchers in this field, and they get satisfaction from knowing they are doing something that is too hard for most other people. Their immune system seems to function better with the result that they become ill less often and are less likely to develop cancer. Certainly they are less likely to develop diabetes and cardiac disease, which is known to be sensitive to diet. Their only complaint is of feeling cold most of the time.

Since the benefits of caloric restriction are mediated through chemical processes in the body, there are many groups currently investigating the possibility of finding the responsible physiological agents. It is thought that an ingredient in red wine may simulate the effects of caloric restriction. There are a number of other similar substances which, if successful, might be able to extend health and longevity in a way analogous to caloric restriction. But we are not there yet.

I agree that a diet which may be very healthy is not going to work if it requires someone to be hungry all the time over the course of a lifetime.

Because of the evidence from many studies of caloric restriction—and other studies—I think the healthiest weight is probably on the lower end of normal. Too thin, though, is not good. Women who are so thin they have stopped menstruating are too thin. It is easy, too, to eat an unbalanced diet in pursuit of thinness. There are all sorts of problems that come from eating foods deficient in one nutritional factor or another. Some studies have suggested that being somewhat thin might actually predispose to illness; but I think these results are explained mostly by the fact that some of the people in these studies started off thin because they were already sick, although not obviously sick.

There are two reasons why I hesitate to recommend that a dieter should aim for being on the thin side:

1. Some people may think I am inadvertently encouraging certain vulnerable individuals to starve themselves. *Anorexia Nervosa* is a

serious, sometimes fatal, condition in which those afflicted want to be thinner and thinner, often to the point where they require hospitalization to ward off starvation. Naturally, I don't want to encourage people to starve themselves. The usual reason why anorexics diet, however, is not to find the exactly right weight, but always to be thinner and thinner. It is the process of dieting, like other compulsive behaviors, that is important to them. Underlying the condition are issues of self-control and also disturbances of body image. That condition, like *bulimia,* which is compulsive binging and purging, is not well-understood, but is not likely to grow out of a normal process of dieting.

2. If dieters start off with the idea that they really need to lose fifty pounds instead of the thirty or forty pounds they had been contemplating, they are likely to feel discouraged and disheartened and possibly likely for that reason to give up before they actually start the diet. The problem here lies in the whole process of setting goals and, in particular, setting the right goals.

THE DISADVANTAGES OF GOAL-DIRECTED BEHAVIOR

I sometimes see in psychotherapy very successful, but very driven, young people who are working very long hours for what seems to me not very clear purposes. I ask them what their goals are— where they want to be 30 or 40 years down the road. Some people, of course, have not really stopped to think about goals. They put one foot in front of the other—they are running in place, really—simply because that is what they have always done. They want to make partner, or get the next promotion, simply because that is what they see immediately in front of them. They run as fast as they can because they are good at it, and because people have always applauded them for being that kind of person.

There are others, however, who have a more subtle and sophisticated response. Initially, they may say only that they want to make a certain number of millions of dollars, or they want to make it to the top of a corporation, or they have some other similarly specific goal; but when I ask them why, they are likely to respond thoughtfully in one of a number of ways:

1. "I want to get to a place where I don't have to worry about money."

2. "I want to reach a certain status where everyone respects me and looks up to me."

3. "I want to achieve enough success that I can do things on my own initiative without requiring the approval of someone else."

Unfortunately, these goals are not achievable. Some people never worry about money and some people always worry about money, and it doesn't matter how much money they have. No one believes this, of course, except very rich people, who know it to be true. Everyone else thinks, if only I had a few thousand or a few hundred thousand dollars more, I would definitely stop worrying about money. But rich people, it turns out, have no trouble imagining some financial calamity or another—and if they worried before they became rich, they continue worrying afterwards. All right, so you don't believe me; it's true, anyway. Secondly, it turns out if you are hugely successful, you move into a community where everyone else is successful; and *no one is impressed!*

Certainly, your children are not impressed. Third of all, no matter how exalted a level someone reaches in a corporation, or in anything else, there is always someone that person has to answer to. Doctors have to answer to their patients (although it doesn't always seem that way); and they have to answer to colleagues for referrals.

Very often, I see these same ambitious people later on in their lives. Sometimes they have achieved their specific goals, and sometimes they haven't; but they are likely to feel unfulfilled and disappointed in either case. Their goals, if they did achieve them, did not bring them the satisfactions they had anticipated. It is what some people have called a mid-life crisis.

This is not to say that it is impossible to be happy. But the happiest people are caught up with the *process* of living, rather than the *goals*. Or to put the matter differently, their proper goals are fulfilled in their day to day existence.

Another example of how misplaced goals spoil things:

A thirty year old woman (or man) is anxious to marry and settle down. In order to find the right person at the right time, however, that woman or man is likely first to have to go on a great many dates with many different people. If that young person sets out on each date expecting to meet the right person, every date is likely to be a disappointment. The trick is to enjoy dating even when it is the wrong person sitting across the table. There are things to do that are fun even if they don't push you immediately to the place where you want to be.

The goals of dieting and losing weight should be measured by the extent that someone has adhered to his or her diet *over the course of a day or a week* and by the exercise that person does *over the course of a day or a week*. What the scale says from day to day is unimportant. Whether or not someone is much closer or only a little closer to losing the weight they need to lose does not matter. On that basis, whether someone has to lose thirty or fifty pounds does not matter. It is the way someone gets to his or her goal that counts in the long run. If the process of dieting can be made palatable (even enjoyable), the dieter will not gain back excessive weight in the future.

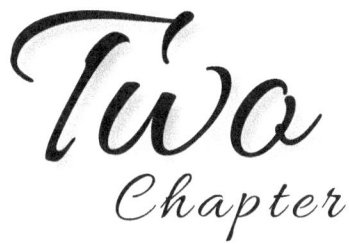

THE CAUSES OF EXCESSIVE WEIGHT OR "HOW DID I GET TO BE FAT WHEN I EAT SO LITTLE?"

*I*t is worth noting that animals do not become obese living in the wild, unless it is in preparation for hibernation or some other anticipated period of fasting. Human beings, on the other hand, have a tendency to get fat; and it looks like we are getting fatter all the time. Our pets have a tendency to get fat. Even the animals we have domesticated for food are fat, at least as fat as we can get them to be. What is different about human beings that allows us to become fat? Were we always inclined to get fat?

Many animals seem to be programmed to eat as much as they can in anticipation that there may not be enough food tomorrow or next week. Probably human beings were always *inclined* to eat as much as they could; they just never had *the opportunity* to eat very much. Food could not have been readily available in prehistoric times, certainly not before agriculture was invented. And then, what food there was spoiled quickly. Also, I have trouble imagining any caveman who was fat surviving the various predators around at that time long enough to reproduce and pass on to his children whatever genes inclined him to become fat in the first place. Really fat people can't run very fast. So, it may be said that people become fat because they now have the opportunity to eat a lot of food. Still, there are more specific theories. It is readily apparent that some of these possible causes of excessive weight overlap:

1. It is thought that some people are destined to gain weight because they have inherited "fat genes" from their parents. There can be no doubt that people vary in their genetic makeup and some people are inclined because of genetic reasons to become tall, or broad-shouldered or squat or fat. It is known, for instance that height is controlled by a number of different genes, probably around twenty. Nevertheless, height is affected also by diet. Fat people tend to come from fat families. That doesn't necessarily mean that they are fat for genetic reasons. They could have learned fat-making behaviors, i.e. eating habits, from their parents when they were growing up. Because of studies of identical twins separated at birth, however, it can be said said, certainly, that there is, indeed, a strong genetic component to body weight. This is not to say that someone so constructed genetically is doomed to becoming fat.

I once saw a woman in her mid- forties who should have been fat, but wasn't. She had two brothers, each of whom weighed over four hundred pounds; and she had a grown child who weighed over three hundred and fifty pounds. Plainly, she had whatever genes it took to get fat. So, I asked her one day, "How come you're not fat?" She explained that she thought it had to do with the fact that she ran for an hour and a half every day before she went to the gym.

2. Diet. The laws of thermodynamics require that the amount of energy that goes into a machine (the human body, for instance) has to balance the amount that goes out; or the extra energy that goes in (food) has to be stored somehow (fat.) So, for *everyone,* no matter what that person's genetic vulnerability, either lowering the food intake or increasing the energy output (exercise) will lower the energy stored as fat. Eating less and less or exercising more and more will cause weight loss. Our modern diet seems to be designed to pack as many calories as possible within the human capacity to eat. High caloric foods seem to be inherently more attractive than other foods for reasons that probably have to do with survival in conditions that human beings found themselves in most of the time throughout our history. But no longer.

Some examples: Chinese who lived in China subsisted on a relatively calorie poor diet and were, for the most part, thin and healthy. Their children, once they came to this country and began eating like the rest of the Americans, became fat in higher numbers and began developing all those illnesses associated with obesity.

There is an Indian tribe that lives in an arid part of the West and has lived there for many generations. (Apparently their land was so unproductive; none of the other tribes were inclined to go to war to evict them.) They survived very well on a very low-calorie diet. When the white men came, however, bringing their accustomed diet with them, the Indians became fat. Now over 90% of them are very fat and approximately the same number suffer from diabetes. They had *evolved* over many generations to live on a sparse diet. Probably the rest of us are similarly not quite evolved enough to cope with our modern diet.

3. Exercise is relevant. A lack of exercise causes obesity; and we are getting better and better at not getting enough exercise. There are exceptions. A whole lot of people are running around, literally, or playing sports, including group sports, at an advanced age. This never used to happen. When I was a kid, if I saw someone running through the streets of Manhattan, I knew they were running for a bus. In particular, it is socially acceptable now for women to play sports throughout their lives. So, there are a minority who are very active physically. But a greater number are less active than people used to be. Television usually gets blamed. Before that there was radio. When telephones first came in, most people thought the device would never catch on. If they wanted to talk to someone, they said, they could just walk over to that person's house. Nowadays, if people really have to go somewhere, they drive rather than walk, use an elevator rather than climb stairs and are, in general, passive rather than active.

Over the long run, physical activity has an effect on maintaining proper weight that is at least as important as a proper diet.

4. Improper eating habits, learned while growing up, are thought to contribute to excessive weight gain over the course of a lifetime. The problem is there is no agreement about what constitutes proper or improper eating habits. Finishing eating everything on your plate used to be considered good; now it is considered bad. You should stop eating when you are no longer hungry. Do not eat that last potato just because it is sitting there on your plate. It is often recommended to dieters that they get in the habit of purposely leaving some food uneaten on their plates.

CONSIDER THESE OTHER RULES OF GOOD TABLE MANNERS:

You should sit down promptly when called to the table and remain seated until everyone finishes eating. Well, sure. We would like our kids to grow up civilized and able to conform their behavior to certain social expectations. But as far as weight control goes, the less time someone spends at the table, the better. Getting up during a meal to do something else for a while is likely to lessen the chance that person will eat something more just to be companionable.

Don't dawdle while eating. Wrong. You should dawdle. Fat people almost always eat too fast. It literally takes a few minutes for the brain to recognize that you have eaten enough. In other words, people will feel hungry for a few minutes even after they have eaten enough. Someone dieting should try to eat slower than the slowest person at the table.

Don't play with your food. Another version of don't dawdle.

Eat your vegetables. Eating vegetables is important. Strict vegetarians hardly ever get fat. And vegetables are healthy in ways that go far beyond maintaining a proper weight. But is it a good idea to hassle kids all the time about eating their vegetables? If eating vegetables, or any other food, becomes an obligation, those foods will become unappealing. I think the best way of encouraging kids to eat their vegetables is to make vegetable dishes that are interesting. If other people in the family eat vegetables, they will too, sooner or later, perhaps a few months or a few years later. No damage will be done in the meantime. In particular, if it is required that if kids are forced to eat their vegetables before getting cookies, they will regard eating vegetables as onerous and eating cookies as a desirable treat. As a reward food.

In general, I think it is a waste of time to try to regulate the proportions of various foods that a child eats. I don't think it can be done.

Just try a little. Encouraging a sullen kid to try a new food is reasonable, I suppose. Every parent does it, even if it inclines the kid in the direction of eating more in general. Actually, I think the effect may be just the opposite. Most sullen kids who are bribed or threatened into trying a new food will not like it as a matter of principle. Besides, saying over and over again "Just try a little. Come on, just a little. You'll like it if you try it. Just take one bite" is annoying; and I think parents should not try to take every opportunity to annoy their kids at the dinner table.

Eat more. Wrong. Some parents have a mistaken idea of how much their child needs to eat to be healthy. Given the opportunity to eat enough, children will eat enough without being encouraged. If a child's weight is in the bottom 25% of kids his age, often the parents will think he is too skinny. Obviously, 25% of normal kids are in the bottom 25% of the weight range for kids their age. If a child is really too thin, which would be very unusual, it is because he is sick in some kind of way; and getting him to eat more will not make him less sick. Very often a child will say she is not hungry during a meal. I don't think it makes sense to threaten her as a way of getting her to eat more. It may be inconvenient to allow her to eat her food a little later on, and maybe it is a reasonable social rule to expect children to eat during meal times, but it is not a good strategy to take from the point of view of encouraging kids to eat only when they are hungry. A more serious problem is a child who is too fat. Rather than restrict his or her diet, which is not likely to work, I recommend some of the measures I mention later on to deal with adult obesity.

<u>Talk less, eat more.</u> Only if you want to encourage a habit of eating more. <u>Don't snack before meals, it will ruin your appetite.</u> It does. It is reasonable, once again, to teach kids to eat at mealtimes, because that is when people usually eat. Still, if your goal is to ruin someone's appetite, it is a good idea to eat a snack before meals; and, later on, I will make that suggestion explicitly.

These various rules suggest that learning how to behave properly when sitting down for a meal may at the same time promote overeating.

Sensible eating habits should be promoted during childhood, assuming we can figure out what is sensible. Plainly, there is an effect these habits have on eating that continues into adult life. Still, I think the effect is less than it is made out to be. Mostly, kids learn all these familiar rules, however out of date or inappropriate they may be, without later on getting fat.

1. Another reason given for gaining weight is <u>too much T.V.</u> The amount of time children watch television has been shown to correlate with weight; the more they watch, the heavier they get. Possibly the effect is through a lack of exercise. Someone sitting inert on a couch is not outside playing ball. Or, perhaps, the food commercials on television that are designed to make them hungry actually do make them hungry.

2. <u>Lack of sleep</u>. People who sleep less eat more. Maybe they have nothing better to do. Maybe there are chemical changes that take place in the brain to compensate for inadequate sleep. There is an appetite center in the brain, and it is known to be affected by circumstances, including, possibly, sleep deprivation.

3. <u>Certain drugs</u>. Some of the anti-depressants, for example, cause weight gain. Over the years I have converted a few chronically depressed, thin women into chubby, but cheery middle-aged women, (although they are not cheery about being chubby.) There are a number of other drugs that act similarly.

4. <u>The sun-spot cycle</u>. As far as I know, there is no correlation between sun-spots and weight gain. I mention this here only to keep the reader's attention.

5. <u>Poverty.</u> Poverty correlates with obesity. There are probably two reasons: there is little access in the inner-city to fresh fruit and vegetables. Processed foods are more fattening. Secondly, healthy foods are more expensive, so, in poor communities, a culture of eating fried foods and other fattening foods has grown up.

6. <u>Certain hormones</u>. The usual "glandular conditions" that are mentioned often by lay people as an explanation for obesity include low thyroid and high cortisone levels. The effects they produce on weight, however, are relatively minor and inconsistent. There are other hormones, however, secreted in the stomach that are known to affect appetite one way or another. Strategies are being

developed to control weight using them; but the results so far have been disappointing. The stomach bypass operations that are used currently to treat morbid obesity are known to affect these hormones, and it may be partially through that mechanism that these operations work.

7. <u>The bacteria that live in the intestine.</u> There are a great many human cells in the body, but ten times that many bacteria take up residence in each of us, particularly in our intestines. These communities of bacteria vary from one person to the next. They help us to digest our food, and some are more efficient at that task than others. Therefore, some people, *given the same amount of food,* absorb more calories than others. So, it is true that a particular person can eat very little, less than other people, and still gain weight. A study was conducted in which a number of people ate the same number of calories and exercised to the same extent; yet there was a perceptible difference in the change of weight each person experienced! There are only three possible reasons why this could happen: for some reason, some people are better at absorbing the calories from their food than others, perhaps because of those bacteria which assist digestion. Secondly, some people are more active *when they are resting (not exercising)* than others. Probably both of these explanations are true. The third reason, an innate difference in metabolism, may result in a somewhat higher body temperature; but the mechanism of this higher metabolism may still come down to moving imperceptibly more than other people.

8. Bacteria affect weight in a second way: they seem to affect the hormones that the stomach secretes to regulate weight. A common cold

virus, adenovirus-36, has been linked to obesity, perhaps because it affects the number of fat cells in the body.

9. <u>The greater availability of food.</u> Over the last 50 years, changing agricultural policies have encouraged more planting of food which then becomes more available. When food becomes cheaper, people eat more.

10. <u>It seems that college students gain an average of one to three pounds during their freshman year.</u> Similarly, men gain a few pounds the first year after they marry. A strategy for avoiding weight gain immediately suggests itself: don't go to college and don't marry.

<u>Also</u>: Obesity has been linked to: stress and/or not enough protein in the diet and/or too much fat in the diet and/or too much carbohydrate in the diet and/or an overly warm house and/or too much light (not enough light causes depression) and/or pollution etc.

It is evident that there are many causes of obesity. They overlap with each other. Perhaps there is a genetic predisposition to have a particular community of intestinal bacteria; and that might in turn affect those hormones that control appetite in a particular way. Recent evidence suggests that exercise changes the effect of the "fat genes." The inclination to exercise itself might be controlled genetically. What matters, I think, is the fact that excessive weight is not simply a failure of will power. It is not a *moral* failing. Dieting has to be approached in a practical way and not with finger wagging.

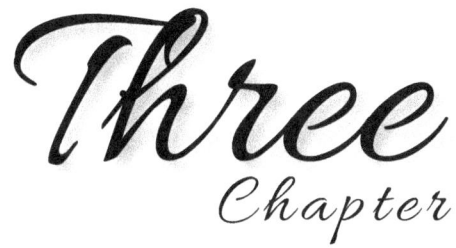

DIETS

*T*he average person who enters a weight loss program weighs slightly more after six months of dieting than at the beginning of the program. This discouraging statistic does not deter most dieters from trying over and over again to lose weight—and typically they do lose weight for a while, only to gain it back relatively quickly. This so-called "yo-yo" dieting is thought to be unhealthy, besides being depressing. It is also frustrating and embarrassing.

Of course, there are men and women who are fat and are comfortable with their appearance and with who they are. But anyone who feels it necessary to enter into a program of dieting starts off feeling dissatisfied with himself or herself. Failure, particularly repeated failures, makes this feeling worse. It is a *public* failure. Fat people may eat secretly to avoid criticism, but they have to present themselves the way they are, fat, or at least thinking they're fat, to everyone all day long. Actually, they look and act pretty much like everyone else. They don't usually stand out as much as they imagine. For one thing there is safety in numbers, and there are very many other fat people. If they are very, very fat, they may avoid going to the theater or even flying on airplanes since they do not fit comfortably in the seats. A few people seem to avoid social situations; but so do others who are not fat. Some have odd habits about clothing. They may wear bulky outfits that they think obscure their weight. Some have wardrobes in different sizes, since they themselves come in different sizes at different times. But it is hard to know, even for a psychiatrist, how people who are fat really feel. Some, I think, have learned to shrug. If being fat is a failing, it is simply one more failing among all the others that they have, and plainly that other people have also. But some others feel bad. They may be especially sensitive to any comments about their appearance. They become defensive in in other ways. Still others feel guilty and ashamed. In general, however, they do not admit to these feelings. They do not complain because they are afraid of the inevitable retort: "Well, then, why don't you lose the weight?" So, I leave it to the imagination, and the personal experience of the reader, to judge what it feels like to be fat.

Whether fat people feel a little bad or a lot, it is plain that many, probably most, are motivated to try over and over again to lose weight. And still they fail. Why?

WHY DIETS FAIL

Diets can fail in the beginning, in the middle, and at the end, and not uncommonly, after the end. Most diets falter even before the beginning.

People put off dieting. Even people who diet on and off for years put off dieting during those times when they are not dieting. They say things like, "I'll diet after the holidays" or "I'll start my diet after the cruise." The implication of this is clear enough, "If I diet, I will not be able to enjoy Thanksgiving. Or the cruise." It is eating, even eating excessively, that defines these experiences. Why? Thanksgiving is a feast, certainly, but it is first of all a family occasion, a time for family to gather together. A cruise is fundamentally a voyage, to be somewhere away from home, and see new things. At least for most people. Put simply, why can't someone diet at these times? The answer, of course, is that dieting—for some—is unpleasant, and so unpleasant that it promises to ruin an otherwise enjoyable experience. To feel this way seems sort of reasonable; but, the fact is, most people can eat moderately on Thanksgiving without feeling deprived. And most people have no trouble passing up the endless supplies of free food on a cruise. Obvious though it may be, it is worth underlining that for people who diet off and on repeatedly, dieting is unpleasant. Dieting is unpleasant in ways that go beyond simply having to eat less of certain favorite foods. The dieter has to wrestle with clothes that don't fit right, and cope with a scale that needs to be jiggled all the time to report a satisfactory weight. Then there is the secret scrutiny of family members who are observing the dieter's progress, or lack of progress.

Some people are leery of Thanksgiving because they feel *they cannot resist food if it is in front of them.* This is a fact that must be dealt with in order to diet successfully.

By the way, if someone says she will begin something after a certain date, such as after New Year's Eve, she will not do it. If doing something really seemed worthwhile to her, she would do it now. Similarly, if a couple tells me they plan on travelling once they retire, I know they will not do it. If they really wanted to travel, they would do it now. The restraints of time and money that they give as explanation for not travelling are not enough to deter other couples in similar circumstances who do travel. Any activity which is put off in the future, even if it seems at first glance to be pleasurable, is put off because it is for some possibly obscure reason upsetting, frightening, or just plain unpleasant.

The people who don't want to diet until after Thanksgiving *do not want to diet,* otherwise they would diet *before* Thanksgiving and, maybe, go off the diet briefly during Thanksgiving. Something that is really worth doing is worth doing now. If it is too hard to do right away, it is worth *starting* to do right now. So, the issue becomes, why don't people wish to start a diet? The answers are not all obvious:

1. Sure, dieting involves giving up something pleasurable. That is easy to see. Everyone understands that. But, really, what the dieter has to give up is only the difference between eating one or two cookies and eating the whole box. On Thanksgiving it is the difference between eating a normal meal and eating a lot, not infrequently to the point of feeling stuffed, sometimes to the point of feeling ill. It is not clear why eating normally, rather than overeating, involves a sacrifice.

2. Dieting means dwelling on the fact of being overweight. Even thinking of dieting spoils eating to some extent. Something similar happens when someone tries to give up smoking. In preparation for their stopping I ask smokers to keep a record of every cigarette they smoke; but if they start to keep records, they stop almost at once. Simply taking note of each cigarette spoils the enjoyment of it.

3. Getting ready to diet, for some people, is like going on a voyage. You can't just start today; you have to get ready first. You have to see the nutritionist, re-join the weight-loss group, make sure the right foods are in the right place and the wrong foods have been removed. This special effort is required to maximize the chance that, once and for all, this time, the diet will work. Often the ordinary business of life, picking up the kids, an extra assignment at work, a visit from the in-laws, interfere and subvert this process. Life being what it is, there is always something going on that gets in the way. If dieting is a voyage, it looks to the dieter like a long voyage.

4. In order to start a diet, the overweight person has to feel there is a reasonable chance of success; and many dieters have good reason to think they will not succeed. Typically, they have failed a number of times before. They tell themselves—and, of course, it is true—that this time might be different; but they have trouble convincing themselves. Which is too bad. Most smokers who finally do stop smoking have failed on an average of eight previous attempts. It is possible to learn something from failure that may make success possible. In order for success to become more likely, however, it is important to proceed in ways that are different than what went before. Most people's inclination is to do the same thing over and over, but try harder this time. Trying the same diet in the same way over and over is a waste of time. Changing the diet by limiting the foods in some new way—only ice cream, only nuts and so on— is not really changing it at all.

The problem: In short, most people fail at dieting before they ever start. They are defeated by the idea that dieting is too difficult and too prolonged, and too unpleasant. And, in the end, unlikely to work.

I think dieting is inherently difficult, but only in the way that changing any habit is difficult.

THE FIRST FEW WEEKS OF A DIET

Usually the first few weeks of the diet go well. The dieter loses weight the first week, perhaps even more than she had anticipated. The exercise goals she had set for herself do not seem onerous. The particular foods she is concentrating on do not seem boring, even if they are not her favorite foods. In a mood of optimism, she may have confided to family or to a few friends that she is actually dieting, thereby risking their disappointment and disapproval if she fails. She is hopeful. The following week, however, the scale indicates that she has not lost any weight. The next week also, or the week after, she has once again failed to demonstrate that she has lost weight, even though she has stayed mostly faithful to the diet and kept, mostly, to her exercise regimen. Now something happens in her life, not directly related to her dieting. Maybe she goes on vacation. Maybe one of the children has gotten sick. Maybe a particularly stressful circumstance has developed at work. Since she realizes that this dieting business is not going to be over as quickly as she hoped, she decides to put it off until this latest complication of life is over. It may be months or years before she starts her diet again. Had she continued to lose weight steadily, these unrelated circumstances in her life would not have caused her to postpone dieting.

The problem: Her expectations were unrealistic. Because her initial weight loss was probably due in part to a loss of fluid, she did not really lose as much weight as she thought. It would be unreasonable to expect that she could continue to lose weight at that rate. It is not even *desirable* to lose weight at a rate faster than one to two pounds a week. Studies suggest that weight lost more precipitously than that usually comes back after the diet is over. The reason, probably, is that that particular diet is too divergent from ordinary eating habits to maintain indefinitely. Putting it differently, weight loss has to extend over a considerable period of time in order to give the dieter enough time to develop a more proper way of eating, by which I mean an interest and delight in eating those healthy foods which do not cause excessive weight gain.

THE MIDDLE OF THE DIET.

Had the person described above been able to persist in her diet and continue to exercise as she had been doing, she might have discovered, nevertheless, that she was no longer losing weight. This tendency to plateau is more common than not. Around this time, also, those friends that have been congratulating her on her loss of weight, are no longer doing so, not because they see that she is no longer losing weight, but simply because they have begun to take her diet for granted. Others haven't even noticed that she has lost weight. Consequently, she becomes discouraged; and it is easy to give up.

The problem: Although the dieter may still be very overweight, prolonged dieting induces the body to go into a "starvation mode." Perversely, the rate of metabolism drops and it takes *more* restriction of calories and/or *more* exercise to cause the same amount of weight loss. It is as if the body has decided that a famine has begun and it would be prudent to start conserving energy. The dieter, herself, feels she is climbing up an endless hill. She doesn't notice any progress, and it seems to her no one else does either.

THE END OF THE DIET (AND AFTER THE END)

Assuming the dieter has the courage and persistence to make those adjustments necessary to continue losing weight, there comes a time when the dieter's weight goals are within reach. Usually she discovers then that she has more weight to lose. The "big bones" she always thought she had, as partial explanation for her weighing a lot, have shrunk along with the rest of her. In other words, she didn't realize just how fat she was. In my experience, someone who has made it this far takes a deep breath and loses the remaining few pounds. She can dress nicely now, and fit into a bathing suit. Now what?

CERTAIN THINGS HAPPEN, OR DON'T HAPPEN:

1. Her family, including her spouse, treat her pretty much the same as they did when she was fat.

2. After an initial burst of enthusiasm, her friends no longer pat her on the back for losing weight. Her children haven't noticed.

3. She was not promoted at work. Strangers have not come into her life clamoring to make friends with her.

4. If she was hypertensive, her blood pressure has dropped some, but she still needs to take medication. If she was diabetic, she is still diabetic, but she takes less medicine, or none at all. She may sleep better. She is healthier; but she doesn't *feel* healthier. The arthritis pain in the back and knees has not gone away.

5. New problems have surfaced. Now that she is at her proper weight, she discovers that she is physically out of proportion. She is skinny in some places and still too fat in others. If she was very fat before, she may have unsightly folds of flesh. Her face seems more wrinkled.

Despite these disappointments, many people feel a lasting sense of accomplishment. They take pride, as they should, in having overcome themselves. But there are others who, after all that effort, feel a sense of let-down; and they are at particular risk of gaining weight again. They don't say to themselves, "I might as well be fat;" but their disappointment makes it more likely that, given a particular temptation— a party, perhaps— they will begin again to overeat—just this one time, they may say to themselves; but soon enough one more time and then again and again.

For these various reasons, and in these various ways, people fail to diet successfully. Another reason is the inclination to rely on fad diets which never offer much hope for dieting successfully in the first place.

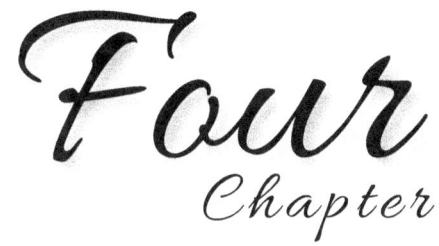

DIETS AND MORE DIETS

*m*any different diets have been promoted for weight loss. Most of them seem to be based on the idea that certain foods control appetite better than others. They are peculiar in the sense that they deviate significantly from an ordinary diet. That is what makes them interesting commercially. They suggest that there is a previously unknown, relatively simple, way of losing weight. They are all ineffective, and some are out and out dangerous. They work, when they do work, by boring the dieter. If you can eat all the ice cream you want, but *only* ice cream, you end up eating less. Even someone who likes ice cream doesn't like it all the time—the same with steak, or eggs, or whatever. Usually, people stick with these narrow diets only briefly and then go back to what they were eating previously. If a diet is narrow enough, and the dieter is stubborn enough, some of the great number of essential nutrients the body requires will inevitably be left out. I have seen a case of pellagra, rare in this country since the turn of the last century, because of a self-imposed dietary restriction. People have died by sticking stringently to diets they considered healthy.

There are other diets marginally less restrictive that have become popular only to be succeeded by another emphasizing an almost opposite approach. There are high fat diets and low fat diets, high carbohydrate diets and low carbohydrate diets. There are high protein diets and low protein diets. Each has a somewhat different rationale. *Each diet has had some success.* I think the reason they succeed, at least for a while, is that they are recommended by enthusiastic and sometimes charismatic proponents, usually in a group setting in which the person dieting receives a lot of attention and support.

Everyone has an emotional stake in making the diet work. And it does. For a while. Keep in mind that a diet that leads to an average weight loss of only ten pounds over the space of six months would be considered wildly successful.

Let us imagine a new diet that is going to be proposed next week by a scientist working secretly in his basement laboratory. It will be called the "Spinach Diet" because it recommends spinach morning, noon and night. And in the afternoon. It is a special spinach that he has grown in the basement with a special light. Let's say this diet works beautifully without turning the dieter green. (Too many carrots turn him orange. Too many tomatoes turn him red. No kidding. Carotonemia, and whatever condition it is you get from eating too many tomatoes, tomatonemia, perhaps, are entirely safe.) The spinach dieter loses weight quickly before he tires of the diet and runs off to the nearest Burger King. He reaches his proper weight. And then what? How does he make the transition to a normal diet without gaining all the weight back?

The problem with all unbalanced diets is that they come to an end, inevitably, without the dieter learning how to eat normal food in the company of normal people. The trick is not to lose the weight, which can be accomplished sometimes by an effort of will, but to keep it off.

There is another diet commonly recommended by doctors and others who recognize the deficiencies of an unbalanced diet: "Eat less." I take this to be a sign of indifference when offered up by a doctor, since the doctor knows the fat person he is talking to cannot, or will not, eat less. Besides, the implication is that the overweight person has been overeating—"pigging out" is the expression one physician used—which may not be the case. Doctors tend to feel frustrated advising obese individuals. They usually comment perfunctorily that their patient should really lose weight, and they give three or four health reasons to do so. Once he has said that a few times, he can think of nothing else to say without seeming to nag. He may recommend a visit to a nutritionist. Actually, psychiatrists have more time than other professionals to talk about these matters; but a referral to a psychiatrist might be construed as insulting. Sooner or later psychiatrists too get to a point where there is nothing else to say. Recently, when I told a woman about some new information about weight-loss surgery, she looked at her watch and said "twenty-five minutes. A new record," meaning that I had gone twenty-five minutes into the session before reminding her that she was fat.

There are some people, of course, who do naturally eat less than others; and they are not fat. But you cannot get to be that kind of person by an effort of will. They naturally feel full, if not stuffed, eating less. Whatever the reason is, it is not because they control themselves better than people who are fat. The same can be said about other indulgences, for that matter. Alcoholism, for example. Most people cannot become alcoholics, *because they feel bad when they have more than two or three drinks.* They have to fight to stay awake. Similarly, some people cannot become fat because eating too much is unpleasant. By the way, I think parents telling their kids they are too fat *over and over again* is a waste of time and likely to spoil their relationship with their children. Kids get fed up with their parents just as overweight people sometimes get fed up with their doctors. This is not to be construed as an endorsement of being fat.

There are other weight loss programs that skip dieting advice; they simply make all the food themselves and deliver it to your door. In such a way, the dieter avoids the pitfalls of deciding for himself what he should eat. Presumably, his judgment is deficient. He would probably be the first to agree. But what happens when the diet comes to an end? How has he learned to eat properly for the rest of his life?

There are other diet programs that have two important elements: dieting in a group context and calorie counting. Similar programs involve prescribing foods or food groups in exact and somewhat arbitrary proportions. In a way, this last group of diets represents another kind of calorie counting.

DIETING AS PART OF A GROUP

For many years psychotherapy has been conducted in a group setting for different kinds of emotional problems. Think of psychotherapy as an attempt to influence a patient to behave in ways that further his own interests but which are likely to make him feel uncomfortable. Often the therapist encourages a patient to be more active and assertive when that is not his natural inclination, for example, looking for a new job, asking someone out for a date, or speaking up at family gatherings. The list is endless. People hesitate to do these things, *which they themselves think they should do,* because they are unsure of themselves or frightened to some extent. Similarly, the therapist is often in the position of discouraging some habitual behaviors which are self-destructive. Examples include demanding or clinging behavior, sulking, chronic tardiness, and gambling. Another endless list. Giving up unhealthy eating habits falls into this group. If psychotherapy is an attempt to influence people to do things which seem contrary to their usual ways, it is easy to see why a group of friendly people, rooting for that person, may have a considerable positive influence on him.

There are a number of commercial programs that rely to some extent on clients entering a group; and there are similar groups of dieters who have come together on their own to help each other. A person enters these diet programs feeling, as do the others in the group, somewhat hopeful, but a little wary and, perhaps pessimistic a little. Often there is someone there who has lost a lot of weight, but for some reason still attends the group. Some of the others have already lost some, but not a lot of, weight; but they are still determined. Some have participated in this exact same program three or four times previously but are persevering still. All of them are welcoming and supportive.

In the following weeks they applaud any weight loss and are sympathetic and understanding when someone has not lost weight, or even, gained a little. A principal message is, "Don't give up. You can do it." Dieters, like everyone else, are motivated by someone rooting for them. They wish to please. During the days between meetings, they try to lose weight not only for themselves, but to please and encourage the others, who are wrestling with their own weight problem. For some people, the group setting makes all the difference.

Still, the same desire to please makes it harder for them to outlast the inevitable periods during which the dieters don't lose weight. They are likely to skip the next meeting because they don't want to disappoint and discourage the others. If they skip a few meetings, they have essentially left the program. The fact that some of these programs have life-time memberships is an indication that by the standard of losing weight *and keeping it off,* they usually fail. But not always. All in all, they have more successes than most of the extreme diets, especially if those other programs are limited to diet alone.

WEIGHING FOOD PORTIONS, COUNTING CALORIES, POINTS, ETC.

There must be more to life than weighing yourself, weighing your food, counting all the calories you eat (thousands) and monitoring aspects of life that usually proceed normally in normal people without anyone consciously directing them. Over the years I have treated people who worried about whether they were urinating the right color, moving their bowels frequently enough, breathing and swallowing normally and sleeping the right amount. All of these bodily functions take care of themselves. I do not want to give them something else to worry about. A proper weight loss diet will merge imperceptibly into a diet that someone can stay on comfortably forever. How is that possible if someone has to spend forever examining his or her food zealously to find the exactly right amount? The circumstances of life are such that people are always eating too much or too little; what matters is whether or not they eat too much over the long run. I don't want someone to feel guilty every time he eats a big dinner.

It is certainly true that high caloric foods, when consumed regularly, incline someone to become fat. *Someone who is already fat should learn to eat less of these foods.* Whatever the rationale of a particular diet, its success will rest on whether or not someone predisposed to become fat for any of the reasons already given will be able to avoid these foods— most of the time, at least. It is not important to know whether a particular portion of food on a particular day is a little bad, or a little worse than that, or pretty bad, really, or very bad. Over the long run counting calories is a distraction. If you set out to walk from New York City to Chicago, you would not need to know just how many feet you travelled each day.

* * *

It would be nice to determine scientifically which of these various diet programs work best; but since the test of a diet takes place over a period of years, measuring success is not practical. None of the diets seem to work obviously better than any of the others. The typical dieter has tried more than one and comes to prefer one more than the others. Certainly, they all work for some people and do not work for most. In every case the diet is likely to work initially when the dieter is most enthusiastic and hopeful and then fail later on. Plainly the point when most people begin to gain weight again is when they begin once again to eat a normal diet. The diet they have been on has not prepared them for eating properly from then on.

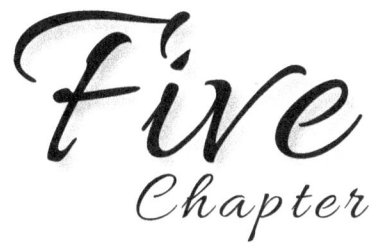

A HEALTHY DIET

There are articles published with some regularity about the health benefits of certain foods and the dangers of certain others. Most of these articles give new reasons for eating foods that we have known for some time are healthful, or still one more reason to avoid foods that have always been suspect. The fact is, we know what we should eat and what we should avoid.

There are a number of metabolic disorders and other conditions that require very special diets. Some of these diets are very familiar. Diabetics should stay away from sugars and starches, which are said to have a high glycemic index, that is, they generate an abnormally high level of sugar in the blood; most hypertensive patients should avoid salt, since salt raises blood volume and blood pressure; patients with certain kinds of kidney disorders should avoid protein; patients with gout should avoid liver and other foods high in purines; patients suffering from celiac disease should avoid gluten, which is present in some grains. It is very important to avoid certain particular proteins in certain inborn metabolic disorders. And so on. I do not presume to recommend a diet for any of these very special problems. The diet suggested below is the best diet for most healthy people, and certainly for most fat people.

Vegetables: Vegetables have to be mentioned first. They contain all kinds of special nutrients (like anti-oxidants and vitamins and other stuff that I won't name because there are too many of them; and I can't keep them straight.) These have health effects that go beyond helping someone to lose weight. Lutein, for example, which is present in leafy vegetables, has been found to lower the risk of macular degeneration, the commonest cause of blindness in the elderly. The cruciferous vegetables: brussels sprouts, cauliflower and broccoli have special benefits, I forget what. Most vegetables (excepting tomatoes) are more helpful raw than cooked since they occupy more space in the stomach and they provide more fiber. Fiber, just to single out one feature of vegetables, lowers cholesterol and may act to prevent colon cancer. (I don't want to emphasize these effects; they are small and controversial. Still, they all act in the same direction: to improve health.) Colored vegetables and fruits, such as blueberries or peppers have a different set of nutrients that are supposed to be especially healthful. I read a report recently that said eating sixteen blueberries every day provided some sort of special benefit. (Every morning I count out the blueberries I put in my cereal. I figure seventeen or eighteen are good too, but fifteen is bad.)

Of course, there are certain vegetables—palm oil, coconut oil, olive oil—which are a form of fat and probably should be avoided for the most part by people who are actively dieting. They are high caloric. When the dieter enters the transition to a more normal diet, small amounts of olive oil are fine. Olive oil leads to a higher level of HDL, the good cholesterol. Substituting olive oil for butter whenever possible is prudent.

I should say something about potatoes. Potatoes are a principal food support for millions of people around the globe. They are a good source of vitamin C and other important nutrients. Diabetics should stay away from potatoes, however, because they have a high glycemic index; that is, when eaten they cause a surge of sugar into the blood. There is some research that suggests that they may also stimulate weight gain in ordinary people out of proportion to their caloric intake, probably for the same reason. Perhaps there is a resultant effect on appetite. The issue is still controversial. This undesirable aspect of eating potatoes seems to go beyond the fact that potatoes are often cooked with fat in foods like potato chips and French fries. Certainly, those foods should be avoided.

That leaves most vegetables. Fruit, in particular, is appealing to most people and is relatively easy to make the centerpiece of a healthy diet. An apple a day goes some distance to keeping the doctor away. (In case it occurs to you someday to save up apple seeds and eat them as you would pumpkin seeds, don't. If you eat enough of the seeds all at once, the cyanide in them is fatal—which is how I know the idea hasn't occurred to you up to now.)

The variety of vegetables available to an American in food stores is just extraordinary. *Being a vegetarian is not a boring experience.* There are some people who are strict vegetarians for moral reasons, but there are others who adhere to this diet because they love the food. If losing weight was the only thing that mattered in the world, I would recommend that everyone become a vegetarian—a veggy-vegetarian. But you have to be careful. For instance, a strict vegetarian may be vitamin B 12 deficient. Ordinarily, however, the typical dieter does not have to concern himself/herself with these considerations.

I sometimes have the fantasy of approaching the Emperor Caligula in his Roman court and offering him a seedless grape, or a tangerine or any of the great number of vegetables he has never heard of, a potato, for instance, and immediately taking a favored seat at his right hand where I could watch him up close while he did all the crazy things he used to do. Forget prosaic stuff like Peacocks' tongues. We eat much better than the Roman Emperors.

By the way, nuts are good for you. They contain trace amounts of essential metals. That's right. You need a certain amount of iron, chromium, copper and other metals to survive. You can eat perfectly well, however, without considering this requirement. Nuts are good, but since they contain fats, too many nuts are not good. Tea and coffee are both reported reliably to have positive health effects, although the matter is still in some dispute in the case of coffee. There is a study that asserts that someone who drinks twenty cups of green tea a day is likely to live longer than someone who drinks only fifteen cups a day; and that person will still likely outlast someone who drinks only ten cups of tea a day. There are laboratory studies that suggest that green tea may prevent cancer from spreading. Like most physicians, I am not readily convinced by one or two, or a half-dozen, studies; but I'm pretty sure that tea is not *bad* for you, so on those days when I don't find it convenient to drink 20 cups of green tea, (every day) I take two capsules of green tea solids.

FISH VS. MEAT

My mother used to tell me that fish was brain food. Almost everything my mother told me about food was wrong; but I read in a medical journal recently that there is some reason to think that fish facilitates and improves brain function. Which goes to show that mothers are not always wrong. There is a theory that human beings separated from more primitive forms of man when they settled along the seashore and survived primarily on fish. It was discovered a number of years ago that Eskimos, who subsist primarily on foods that contain very large amounts of fish oil, had a very low incidence of heart disease. Immediately, other people started ingesting huge amounts of fish oil, with the result that they started bleeding uncontrollably. These people had not evolved to subsist solely on fish. Fish oil is probably good for most people, but only in the right amounts. This is one example of a basic nutritional fact: *Whether a particular food is good for you or bad for you depends on the amount that you eat.* Even water, when taken in prodigious amounts, is bad for you. I have taken care of two individuals who developed a paranoid psychosis after drinking too much water.

The effects of fish oil, like many other foods, are complicated. It interferes with blood clotting, which is a good thing when the aim is to prevent blood clots in the coronary arteries. If you already have a tendency to bleed, it is obviously a bad thing. It also can substitute for other fatty acids in arachidonic acid, which is a substrate for inflammation. It has been used, therefore, in attempts to cut down the inflammation in various arthritic conditions. This was a reasonable hypothesis, which turned out, like so many other good ideas in medicine, not to work very well. Fish oil has been used to prevent depression. Since no one wants to invest two or three hundred million dollars to prove whether fish oil really works in this way, no one knows for sure. There is epidemiological evidence, in any case, that suggests strongly that eating fish correlates with longevity and good health. For that reason, I think it is fair to say, *eating fish is good for you.* I should say in passing that certain fish tend to accumulate mercury, and, therefore, eating A LOT of deep sea fish—salmon or tuna—may be bad for you.

There is a different anthropological theory that suggests that human beings separated from more primitive forms when they began eating meat. Meat has lots of calories, and, so the story goes, people had more energy for doing human-type things, making beads, drawing pictures, and, in general, acting like modern human beings. Actually, you have to go back a long, long way to reach a time before humans began eating meat. Human beings have always eaten pretty much any animal in the vicinity, the bigger the better. Bands of prehistoric people relocated from time to time to different continents; as soon as they got there oversized animals—woolly mammoths, the Moa, giant sloths and so on—died out. We have hunted these and many other animals to extinction.

Meat is a favored food wherever it is available. Historically, or prehistorically, we used to run down our food, antelopes, for instance, if you can believe that, because it was important to eat high caloric meat in order to give us enough energy the next day to run down more antelopes. Meat is eaten everywhere now, although some of these foods seem strange to us: horses, dogs, slugs and so on. The choice is not between "white meats" such as pork or chicken and "red meats" like cows and deer; there are also insects. It turns out insects are very nutritious and valuable. Termite mounds in certain areas of Africa are passed down from one generation to the next. All these meats vary in protein and fat content and in calories. Cooking them one way or another may have certain advantages or disadvantages; but I am disinclined to recommend one kind of meat over the other. They are not that different. Besides, if I were to recommend insects, which are in fact recommended by some authorities on insects, you would not pay any attention. It is important to note in this connection that tastes in food are a cultural phenomenon. Italians like pasta because they were brought up eating pasta. Japanese like sushi for the same reason. *But these food preferences can change.* If one food is unavailable, people begin to prefer foods that are available. When I was told unexpectedly that I had coronary heart disease and had to eat less meat, I began eating sushi, which initially seemed distasteful to me, especially its texture. I grew to love it.

A patient of mine who was dieting successfully told me that the beef stew he used to look forward to was now "disgusting" to him.

Since no one has to run after antelopes any more, it is not necessary to eat high caloric foods. I think a reasonable attitude towards eating meat was expressed by Thomas Jefferson, who said meat should be used as a condiment, that is, as a flavoring for other foods.

I know what the reader's reaction is to this idea:

1. I like meat

2. I can't imagine not liking meat.

3. A little bit of steak would just leave me wanting more.

Meat is a perfectly satisfactory food, but eating meat in excessive amounts encourages weight gain. One of the positions I take in this book is that *it is possible to eat meat, or any other food, in portions that do not encourage weight gain, and that are satisfying, nevertheless.*

In summary: more fish, less meat.

Alcohol, Vitamins, Herbs, and Other Stuff

I don't think any of these substances have much relevance to a weight-control diet; but I sort of feel obligated to say something about them anyway.

Alcohol: Alcohol is another example of a food which is good in certain amounts and bad in greater amounts. One drink a day, a glass of wine, perhaps, raises the good cholesterol (HDL) much more than exercise, which also raises it somewhat. Other positive effects are reported from time to time. Epidemiological evidence suggests that limited amounts of alcohol affect health favorably and may increase longevity. Three drinks or more have the opposite effect. Alcoholics, as everyone knows, are very unhealthy in many ways. They have gastric disease, liver disease, neurological diseases and psychiatric diseases—two different kinds of psychosis: Korsakoff's psychosis, a confabulatory condition which I won't explain; but it's not good, and Wernicke's psychosis, which, among other things, involves paralysis of eye muscles. Someone who is an alcoholic should never drink. Alcoholics who have one drink lose all restraint and cannot resist drinking more. (Don't compare this to someone who eats a piece of chocolate cake and then goes on to eat the whole thing. Alcohol inhibits areas of the brain which are associated with impulse control. For that reason, cocaine users are much more likely to get high if they have had a drink first. Someone who eats a whole chocolate cake, and, of course, I know people who have done this, are making some sort of obscure point. Certainly, no one is hungry enough to eat a whole cake.)

Dieters should understand that alcohol has a significant amount of calories.

Vitamins:

The medical profession has usually taken the stance that sufficient vitamins are present in an ordinary healthful diet so that taking supplements are unnecessary. In part they are responding to false and sometimes outlandish claims by the huge, unregulated industry that manufactures these products. This is still a controversial issue. I recently read a medical article suggesting that supplements may not only be not helpful, they may be out and out dangerous.

On the basis of the bulk of evidence available currently, I think there is a place for taking vitamin supplements. In the first place, many people do not eat a balanced, healthful diet; and, secondly, as people age, they absorb vitamins less efficiently. There are minerals, such as iron, that should not be taken as supplements unless the person has a documented iron deficiency. Iron may act as a carcinogen and creates other health problems; and there are other vitamins and nutrients that can be taken in doses so high that they become hazardous; but there are many people walking around that have subtle, but important, deficiencies that are correctible by taking supplements.

Vitamin D is an example. Until recently Vitamin D was thought to be important only to prevent rickets, which is a bone disease. We now know that Vitamin D is important in maintaining immune function, cardiac function and probably a normal mood. The further north someone lives, the more likely that person is to be vitamin D deficient since the vitamin is produced in the body by sunlight. In this time of using sunblock, practically everyone is vitamin D deficient. (There is still some debate, however, about exactly what level of Vitamin D is best. It is theoretically possible to take too much.)

The National Institutes of Health come out with recommendations in this regard, but they are not entirely trustworthy. *They do not want ever to have to rescind their recommendations;* therefore, they hesitate to make specific recommendations until they are absolutely sure they are right. As a consequence, for instance, they postponed recommending adding folic acid to our food until years after it was obviously a sensible precaution against pregnant women giving birth to babies with certain deformities. If they had taken the opposite approach with beta carotene, for instance, they would have risked having recommended it, only to withdraw that recommendation later on when it turned out that beta carotene fosters lung cancers under certain circumstances. For myself, and my patients, I think it is reasonable to go by current evidence, even if in the future further evidence suggests that what seems right now will turn out to be wrong.

I do not think taking vitamins bears directly on the issue of losing weight except that certain extreme diets must be supplemented in this way.

<u>Salt</u>

The amount of salt in a typical diet varies to a great extent not only from individual to individual, but also from country to country. The recommendation from public health authorities, although still controversial, has always been to minimize salt intake. If everyone cuts down on salt, there is a noticeable decrease in the incidence of hypertension and in those cardio-vascular diseases that are secondary to hypertension. This is a phenomenon that takes place only over a period of years. And there are many people who are not salt sensitive. Over a range of hours and days, the body responds to a greater than usual salt intake by retaining fluid. In time the kidney excretes the extra salt and fluid and the apparent weight gain evaporates. *It is important that the dieter realizes that his/her weight can bounce around like this without affecting long range weight control.* Using less salt leads over time to wanting less salt. That is, the taste buds adjust to a lower level of salt. My suggestion is that dieters who do not have a specific recommendation to the contrary from their physicians ignore the question of salt altogether, at least until someone enters upon a maintenance diet. There are enough adjustments to make initially without looking for more.

<u>Sugar</u>

People are eating more and more sugar. The increasing use of sugar seems to parallel the increasing incidence of obesity and diabetes. Although the mechanisms by which sugar is metabolized are not entirely known, the consensus view is that it promotes these conditions and others. Certain drugs, including the anti-depressants, specifically stimulate an appetite for sweet foods, such as candy. Sugar is very bad for diabetics. It is high caloric and should be used sparingly by everyone else. Some authorities think sugar is addicting and, therefore, using it inclines someone to use it more and more. For the same reason, it may be difficult to stop using sugar all at once. I think sugar, like all the other foods described in this book, can be used safely in moderation.

Herbs

Herbs have always been used in cooking; and that's great. Many of the recipes offered further on in this book will depend on herbs to make them interesting and varied. However, other herbs are sold now as a "natural" substitute for drugs. Although it is illegal to make claims for their curing mental or other medical diseases, they are sold, nevertheless, plainly for those purposes. I strongly recommend that people do not use these products! These are some of the reasons:

1. Although some of them have been used for thousands of years, these same agents, many of them, are toxic to the liver or kidneys and have been killing people for thousands of years.

2. The F.D.A. cannot oversee the sale of these agents unless they have been shown clearly to have injured people. (Some ephedrine-like herbs have been taken off the market for this reason, but not before many people got sick.)

3. Although most of the substances have no effect, some of them have considerable effects and may interfere with other drugs the patient may be taking, such as certain anti-depressants or anti-cancer agents. Sometimes the combination is deadly.

4. Although the label on a bottle of herbs states that the bottle contains a particular substance, there is no requirement that it actually does. Often it does not. When it does, there is no guarantee that the amount of the substance is as it is represented to be. Active ingredients vary from manufacturer to manufacturer and batch to batch.

5. These products are often adulterated purposely with active psychotropic drugs, such as the Valium family of drugs, so that they will have a noticeable effect.

Some suspicious people think the drug companies are out to poison the population in order to make more money. These companies have proven careless in the past, and, certainly, they are motivated by making money; but it is not in their interest to have to pay out billions of dollars in damages when they sell a product that turns out to be harmful. Typically, hundreds of millions of dollars have been spent testing and bringing a new drug to market. On the other hand, there is no law requiring that herbs be tested in this way; and it is not in the manufacturers' interest to do so. Most herbs sold in health food stores do not promote health; and some are dangerous.

<u>Drugs</u>

Certain drugs have been used to lessen appetite or to interfere with the absorption of fats from the intestines. They haven't worked very well. Those that do work to some extent, such as the amphetamines, have proven dangerous; and they do not usually lead to much weight loss in the first place. Other drugs that cut down appetite have been taken off the market because they tend to cause depression or certain cardiac disturbances. The drugs that affect absorption of fat often cause diarrhea; and they too are not very effective. Even when it seems that these drugs are working, they are likely to stop working after a while. Remember, the goal of dieting is not to lose weight, but to achieve a stable weight from then on. No one thinks these drugs should be used indefinitely. I think it is possible, even likely, that someday appetite suppressants that are safe will become available. New drugs are in the process right now of being approved, but past experience suggests that they cannot form the basis for long-term successful dieting.

* * *

The diet suggested above—more fresh vegetables, more fish, less meat—has been recommended for all kinds of purposes: preventing heart disease, stroke, Alzheimer's disease, cancer, diabetes and so on. Highly saturated fats, processed foods, and sucrose (sugars) are bad, always with the caveat that a little of one of these "bad" foods is okay "Good" foods, besides being healthy, are less likely to make you gain weight, the "bad" foods work in the opposite way. Someone might discover a new fruit that has an especially good combination of anti-oxidants, or some other such thing; but I think that our understanding of what constitutes a proper, healthy diet is not going to change with time. To say that pomegranates are better or worse than tomatoes is to miss the point. There are very many interesting, even exciting, vegetables and fruits. Staying on a healthy maintenance diet is like traveling downstream on a boat. You can move around comfortably and sit in one place or another; you just can't jump over the side.

How to Eat

Knowing what to eat is straightforward, knowing *how* to eat is another matter. Fat people tend to eat differently than other people, at different times and in different amounts. They have different eating habits and their expectations about eating, weight loss and exercising are all different. In certain ways they are ill-informed. To start with, they think a normal diet is *much more* than it really is. They may think they are eating small amounts, or, in any case, what others are eating, when, in fact, they are eating more.

Eating in restaurants could easily mislead someone about how much a person is supposed to eat. If someone judged by a typical menu, a diner is expected to eat an appetizer, an entrée and a dessert, along with an alcoholic drink, perhaps, and bread and butter, and olives. No one could eat that much regularly without getting fat. And on certain formal occasions, there might be other courses offered also. A dieter might well think that if she eats only an appetizer and an entrée she is dieting! Some of these meals may be over 2500 or even 3000 calories. A typical dieter may limit herself to 1500 or 1600 calories a day, and some people need to eat as few as nine hundred or a thousand calories a day to be able to lose weight successfully. Just as an alcoholic should avoid bars when he first becomes sober, a dieter should consider avoiding elaborate (long) meals in restaurants. And, as in the case of alcoholics, this strategy should only be for a while. The goal for a successful dieter is to eat in the company of other people without feeling deprived or tempted to eat excessively. Dieters have to start with a proper appreciation of how little food it takes to eat enough.

A principal reason dieters become discouraged is that they start with unrealistic expectations. They need to know if the diet they are starting is strict enough to work! Otherwise, they will see little evidence that it is working, and they will become discouraged..

Some dieters have the idea that certain foods "burn fat" more than others. This is not true. They may think that eating at certain times of day is better, or worse, than at other times. This is not true. They may think that drinking a lot of water cuts down on appetite. This is not true, but for a particular reason: water is absorbed directly through the stomach and will not cause someone to feel full for any length of time. The misconceptions dieters, and people in general, for that matter, have about food are legion. Here are some facts:

1. An amount of food eaten during the course of four or five or six meals will cause less weight gain than that same amount eaten in two or three meals. The process of digestion costs energy. Eating a lot of food all at once is more efficient, from the point of view of conserving energy (absorbing more calories.) I have known a man who ate only one meal a day for years and still lost weight and maintained that weight loss; but he was an exception. Most ordinary people eat something all day long. I eat breakfast, a small snack during the morning, a small lunch, commonly something during the afternoon, a small dinner and a couple of snacks during the evening and night. I am almost never hungry, (particularly during meals.)

2. What is enough food for one person is not likely to be enough for someone else. Big, very active people need more calories. Most people who eat as little as I do would be hungry. If someone is dieting for over a month and has not lost weight, the amount of food he has been eating is too much, or he is exercising too little. If someone else is losing weight on what seems like a considerable amount of food, he is not eating too much. It may well be, for reasons that

have been described above, that successful dieting involves eating less than someone else who is just as active.

3. Binge eating is not due to being hungry. Some examples: A woman who has eaten very little all day decides after dinner to go to a grocery store and buy a box of cookies. She proceeds to eat the whole box. When asked why, she said she felt depressed and eating made her feel better. She gave no explanation why it was necessary to eat the whole box of cookies. She has been binging in such a way most of her life. She does not throw up after eating, as some others do, to prevent weight gain.

Interesting questions: Why does stuffing herself with a desirable food make her feel less depressed? We have heard people say this sort of thing so often, it seems to make sense; but I think most people who have eaten a lot do not feel a difference in mood. They simply feel full (not hungry.) A common explanation is that cookies are a "reward food," but why can't this person choose a reward of a different sort? She complains bitterly about being fat. A possible reason might be that this self-indulgent practice brings with it its own punishment. Perhaps the dieter *wants* to punish herself. (I hate explanations of this sort.) Please note that this was not impulsive eating. She set out to buy cookies in order to binge.

Another example: A man wakes up in the middle of the night, most nights, and binges. Later on, in the morning, he thinks he may have been hungry, but he doesn't remember very well. He prefers certain foods to others, but will eat anything in the refrigerator. He gains weight, but not very much. He eats normally during the day. There are others who are similarly compulsive night eaters. Some researchers think this habit may be due to a subtle disturbance of brain function; but if it is, it is subtle, indeed. No neurological signs are evident.

Another example: A young, obese woman quarreled with her room-mate who then asked her to stay away from a party she was giving for her friends. Instead, the young woman snuck into the kitchen and ate a whole birthday cake that had been expected to serve eight people. This particular kind of bingeing I understood. It was eating as revenge. She used to enjoy crowding other people when she sat on a bus.

Still another example: A still relatively young man frequently went out eating with friends and took pride in being able to out-eat everyone else. Peculiar, but once again, not hard to understand. People take pride in almost anything. At one point I entered contests in which I could demonstrate that I could write smaller than anyone else.

A much more characteristic example: A young overweight woman ate three chocolate bars *before* visiting her home where she expected to be served her favorite, although fattening, meal. Since she knew she would be going off her diet anyway, she felt she might as well gorge herself. She set out to overeat.

Very often, if a dieter who has eaten something he/she feels is fattening, that person will then figure, what the hell, I might as well eat the whole thing.

The first time I heard anyone speak this way, I was startled. It seemed to me that person was saying that having shot himself in the foot, he might as well go ahead and shoot himself in the knee. But, the fact is, this is a common psychological mechanism that shows up in many different contexts, in any situation in which someone is doing something that person enjoys doing but thinks is wrong.

Examples: Someone buys marijuana to use just a little at a time, but finds she cannot stop smoking it until it is all gone.

A gambler decides to wager only a particular amount, for fun, but then decides to bet more and more until he has no money left.

Someone decides to put off working for a few hours to play ball, and then plays ball all day long without ever getting back to work.

In order for a diet to be successful, a strategy has to be developed for dealing with this tendency to lose all restraint after having gone off the diet just a little. It leads not only to binging, but to giving up the diet altogether.

The following chapters give psychological strategies for dealing with the various, characteristic problems associated with dieting and maintaining a proper weight.

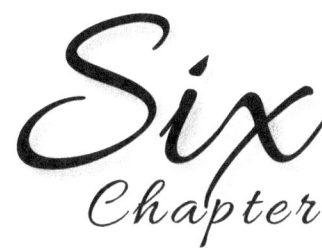

Six
Chapter

EXERCISE!

I think I should probably write this whole section in capital letters. Even before talking about eating the right foods in the right ways, I want to emphasize exercising properly. Although over the short range, dieting stringently has a more obvious effect on weight loss, over the long run exercise has a more profound effect. There are people who eat inordinate amounts of foods and maintain a proper weight nevertheless, because they are very active. Probably, human beings have evolved to eat as much as possible and exercise all day long. Almost all the people I have known who have lost weight successfully and kept it off have maintained a life-long habit of exercise. Dieters become dissatisfied with the effects of exercising only because they expect too much from too little effort! Imagine that someone with a strep throat was told to take penicillin three times a day. On his own initiative that patient decides that one pill is enough. When he fails to improve, he decides that penicillin doesn't work! The typical person who exercises as part of a weight control program does something similar. Someone who thinks a little bit of exercising is okay, or, at least, better than nothing, is going to be disappointed with the effect of exercise.

It is said that fifteen minutes of brisk walking a day helps cardiac function. Possibly it does; although I think that would be difficult to determine exactly. There is even some highly debatable research that suggests small amounts of exercise like this may lessen the effect of the "fat genes." But the requirements for real weight loss are much more. Experience suggests that in order for exercise to contribute meaningfully to weight loss, someone has to exercise aerobically for at least 45 minutes to an hour and at least four to five times a week. Walking the dog does not count! Cleaning the house does not count! Being on your feet all day long does not count! What relatively prolonged exercise accomplishes is that it speeds up metabolism to a certain extent for the rest of the day. You have probably heard that bicycling for a half- hour burns up the calories in a single cookie. That is beside the point. Significant exercise acts in a way similar to turning up the thermostat. People become literally warmer. Weight-lifting and other intermittent exercises do not seem to work as well as steady aerobic exercise. Similarly, swimming does not work as well as running because the body tends to be cooled by the water rather than heating up. I have known only one person who lost weight successfully by swimming; and he swam for about an hour and fifteen minutes every day.

I know that the amount of exercise I am recommending is way more than the average person gets in our sedentary culture. I understand that the typical reader of these pages will immediately think that he/she doesn't have the time for this much exercise, let alone the inclination.

Two anecdotes: I saw a patient who had just been divorced. Her husband left her and left the country at the same time. She had to take care of three children under the age of six by herself. She had a full-time job and was looking for another job that paid more. As most people understand, looking for a job is a full-time job in itself. She spent considerable time interviewing babysitters for her children. She saw her parents once a week and she was actively starting to date. She also went to the gym three times a week. I asked her how in the world she found time to go to the gym given her busy schedule. She looked at me as if I had asked a foolish question; and, perhaps, I had.

"Exercising is very important to me," she replied. When something is very important to you, you find time to do it.

The second anecdote concerns me. At the age of 49 I developed coronary heart disease. I had spent the previous 25 years sitting in a chair talking to people; but suddenly I had to exercise. I believed my life depended on it. I did not want to die with my children still not grown up. Despite working over fifty hours a week, writing books and doing all the things being in a family requires, I started jogging for an hour a day, seven days a week. I found time to do it because I felt I had to! As a consequence, two other things happened: although I had been my proper weight (what I weighed when I graduated high school) I began to lose weight, without trying. I was five foot, nine inches tall and I dropped from 151 pounds to 137. Although I was, after a while, probably in the best shape of my life, people began to look at me askance and ask if I was okay. I remember these figures because around that time I read of another physician who was running marathons and was my height. He weighed 127 pounds! People who are exercising properly are probably at the low end of the normal weight range.

I want to emphasize the second thing that happened to me: I began to like jogging! It took, as I remember, two to three months; but physical activity that was simply a chore to me at the beginning began to be fun. I think if someone had asked me, I would not have believed at first that I could enjoy the everyday, unchanging routine of jogging, but I did.

As a psychotherapist, I struggle every day to convince people that they can change in certain ways without having to turn into a different human being. They can grow to like things they did not like initially. They can become accustomed to doing things that have always frightened them. They can grow.

People think of themselves as being poured out of a mold. "This is the way I am. This is the way I have always been. This is what I like. I am not going to do these particular things, because that is not the kind of person I am." People want to feel better, but they don't want to behave any differently than they have in the past. Or, probably more accurately, they don't think they can. Other people can do these ordinary things, which they may very well recognize would be advantageous to them, but they can't. And that's that. They won't exercise properly because they just can't see themselves doing that. Dieting properly also requires long-term, permanent change of just the sort we have been talking about. People can imagine themselves dieting for a while, but they have trouble imagining that they will eat differently permanently.

In a way it is easy to understand why someone has trouble giving up something that it seems to them they have always enjoyed, and will always want to enjoy; but the truth is *any change at all* is hard for people.

Example: People come to me sometimes because of sleeping problems. I make a number of recommendations, one of which is to turn the clock to the wall during the night. Strangely, people sleep more than they realize. They look at the clock at 2 A.M., 2:10 A.M, and 2:20 A.M. and do not realize that they have been sleeping during the intervening moments. Each time they look at the clock they get upset. They worry about not sleeping enough, and, getting upset tends to wake them up more. There is no reason to know the time in the middle of the night. No one has ever been able to give me a good reason for knowing the time in the middle of the night; yet everyone has a hard time breaking this habit. It is not that patients *enjoy* checking the time. The opposite is true. Yet typically, it takes me *weeks* to get someone to turn the clock to the wall. (They turn it a little to the wall. They move the clock a few feet further away; but they don't acknowledge the fact that they are not supposed to know the time or want to know the time.) Sooner or later, I can usually get them to go along with this relatively minor change of habit, sometimes with dramatically positive results. But there are a few patients who angrily refuse. "I *got* to know what time it is," one patient said, before storming out of my office. It is as if any change at all is a violation of that person's understanding of himself.

Since I have spent most of my professional life dealing with the anxiety disorders, I have spent most of my time trying to motivate patients into confronting their fears. These fears are always unrealistic; otherwise they would not be construed as implying a disorder. Naturally, there are ways that this can be accomplished: a little bit at a time, with helpers, proper preparation, etc. In the end, motivating such people always involves convincing them of two things: the bad consequences of *not* confronting their fears and the certainty of becoming less afraid if they do. If they don't confront their fears, they usually become worse. If they do confront them, they become less afraid. Put a different way, therapy involves convincing people to try new things and new ways of behaving long enough to see that what I tell them will happen actually will happen. Their previous experience suggests that I am wrong. They have not had the experience of growing less afraid, for instance; so they don't believe me. The reason is that *this process*

65

takes a period of time. Someone who wishes to overcome a fear of elevators has to spend a lot of time in elevators. So, that's the trick.

Someone who thinks he/she will not enjoy exercising, or enjoy eating a different diet, has to be persuaded to try these things long enough for those changes to take place. In the case of exercise, I think that person should expect to exercise regularly for a matter of a few months before exercise becomes enjoyable. But it will! Running and jumping are the kinds of things animals, particularly primates, enjoy. Monkeys are bouncing around all day long because that is what they like doing, not because someone told them that jumping around was good for them. Humans will enjoy these activities if given a chance. Look at the proliferation of health clubs and the numbers of people who jog regularly. Of course, certain kinds of exercise are fun right from the beginning. These are sports for the most part. Aerobic sports include tennis, racquet ball, basketball and bicycling. Not golf. Certain activities, (swimming laps, for instance— which I do now since I developed a bad back after previously jogging for twenty years) are inherently less interesting; but even these become satisfying after a while.

By the way, the time problem always solves itself because anything done routinely seems to take less and less time.

Exercise has health benefits that go much further than maintaining a proper weight. There is good evidence that exercise minimizes the risk of diabetes (in ways not associated just with weight loss), lessens the risk of heart attacks and stroke and cancer, increases longevity, and perhaps most important of all, significantly reduces the risk of Alzheimer's disease. I recommend exercise to patients with a history of depression. There is evidence that it prevents the depression from returning.

<u>Proper Dieting.</u>

IT IS NOT POSSIBLE TO DIET CONTINUOUSLY OVER THE COURSE OF A LIFETIME! IT IS NOT POSSIBLE TO MAINTAIN A PROPER WEIGHT FOREVER BY AN EFFORT OF WILL ALONE! IT IS NOT POSSIBLE TO GO THROUGH LIFE HUNGRY!

It is also not possible to eat high caloric foods if you already feel stuffed by having previously eaten a lot of low caloric foods. The goal of proper dieting is to substitute low-caloric (low density) foods for those that are responsible for making you fat. WHENEVER YOU ARE HUNGRY, YOU SHOULD STUFF YOURSELF WITH THESE FOODS! Even those binge eaters who claim they eat even when they are not hungry will be unable to eat more if they stuff themselves with these foods. This strategy is a special case of what is known more generally as Preemptive Action, an important element of psychotherapy.

PREEMPTIVE ACTION

I wrote previously of the purpose of psychotherapy, which, speaking broadly, is to help patients get to where they want to go in life. Each person has particular strengths and weaknesses, not to mention symptoms, which make the process subtle; but the recurrent, overriding problems of psychotherapy are two: sometimes patients realize only after a period of time that the place they really want to get to, or their goal, is different from what they thought they wanted. For instance, someone may strive to be a movie star, when what they really want is recognition from certain important people in their lives. The second problem is that, invariably, getting to that goal requires their doing things that are uncomfortable and anxiety-provoking. Otherwise, they would have made those changes on their own initiative long ago. Maybe they need to be more assertive or more willing to risk entering into a new relationship or more willing to do any of a hundred other things. Part of that effort is often the need to *refrain* from doing certain accustomed, self-destructive behaviors. These behaviors can involve any aspect of their lives. Because they are habitual and difficult to stop, they seem impulsive. *The patient seems not to be able to stop them although he/she sees clearly that stopping them is desirable.*

Some examples of these harmful activities:

1. Alcohol and drug abuse.

2. Violent behaviors.

3. Clinging and demanding behaviors.

4. Promiscuity and philandering

5. Avoidance behavior

6. Making jealous accusations.

7. Compulsive gambling or shopping

8. Overeating.

This list can be expanded indefinitely. Dealing with these self-defeating behaviors and the problems that grow out of them takes up most of a therapist's time.

One way to refrain from these activities is by taking preemptive action. A preemptive action is a behavior which interferes with, or prevents, some other undesirable behavior. It is easier to perform a preventive action than *not* do a self-destructive behavior by an effort of will alone. An example: alcoholics who have demonstrated over time that they cannot resist impulsively taking a drink may agree to take Antabuse each morning. Antabuse is a drug that interacts strongly with alcohol. They are then simply *unable* to take a drink for the rest of the day, since if they do, they will become violently ill.

An example from mythology: The Sirens were women, perhaps three or four, maybe even five, but at least two, with unpronounceable names, who endangered shipping in the Mediterranean by singing seductive, sweet, but sad, songs that so captivated sailors that they jumped into the water and drowned or cracked up their vessels on some nearby rocks. According to Homer, Odysseus prevented this calamity by having his crew tie him to the ship's mast so that he could not be lured to his doom. In a different story, Jason of the Argonauts overcame the same danger by having Orpheus sing a song loud enough and sweet enough to make inaudible the Siren's song.

Other examples drawn from everyday life:

1. Someone trying to stop smoking jumps in the shower whenever he has the urge to light up a cigarette. Even people who smoke everywhere cannot, or will not, smoke in the shower.

2. Someone inclined to get in bar fights, decides to avoid bars.

3. A patient who washes his hands compulsively so often that they have developed fungal infections is brought into the hospital and

kept in a room where there are no faucets or other means for him to wash his hands.

4. A cocaine user moves out of his neighborhood to avoid accustomed places or people he associates with his drug use. Similarly, a woman trying to stop using marijuana goes on a cruise where she knows the drug will be unavailable.

5. A compulsive shopper tears up her credit cards.

6. A clinging and demanding woman finds herself calling her ex-boyfriend repeatedly although he has asked her to stop. She knows these repeated phone calls make the chance of reconciliation less likely. To prevent herself from calling him impulsively, she spends as much time as possible at work or with friends.

7. A woman afraid of pigeons and inclined to run away learns to run *at* them instead.

8. A man with health anxiety takes his pulse all day long. He knows this makes his preoccupation with health worse, but he finds it impossible to stop. Finally, he asks his wife to stop him when she sees him doing this.

9. Someone who needs to jog for health reasons finds himself stopping prematurely. Instead of jogging on a machine in his house, he jogs away from his house, guaranteeing that he has to jog all the way back.

These preemptive actions are most typically something that simply prevents some other action from taking place, for example, a compulsive shopper tearing up her credit cards. Or Odysseus having himself lashed to a mast. A better approach, when it is possible, is to have the undesirable, but more or less irresistible, behavior replaced by a different, but satisfying, activity. Jason's strategy of having the Sirens' song replaced by Orpheus's song is for that reason a better solution to the problem of the Sirens' appeal.

One example of this strategy in the management of narcotic addiction is the use of Methadone, another narcotic, but one less likely to cause a high. The use of Methadone, which produces some of the same effects, but much less, allows the addict to resist using heroin and, therefore, live a more or less ordinary life.

Habitual overeating is a good example of a behavior which the individual recognizes as being bad for him/her, but which that person seems, nevertheless, unable to stop. Since overeating can be carried to such an extreme that it causes morbid obesity and an immediate threat to life, radical preemptive actions have been tried, including wiring the jaws shut! If the goal of dieting is to lose weight, this works. The obese person eats (drinks) a little through a straw. And loses weight. The problems with this approach are obvious:

1. What happens when the jaws are unwired? There has been no opportunity for the obese person to learn how to eat normally, under normal conditions, experiencing the same temptations to overeat that led to the problem in the first place.

2. Not many people are willing to have their jaws wired shut.

The principal problem implementing a successful program of preemptive action is that people resist changing their habits and undertaking _any_ change in the way they manage their impulsive behavior. Radical treatments such as wiring their jaws shut are likely to be dismissed out of hand.

A more effective way of dealing with morbid obesity is the various operative procedures that serve to diminish the stomach's capacity to hold food. These are bypass surgery and banding procedures. The effect of these interventions is complicated and subtle. To some extent they lessen the person's hunger along with decreasing his ability to eat to excess. Like other operations, they are not without risk, but they are in some instances immediately life-saving; and in many other cases they obviously diminish the risk to health long run. Diabetes can be reversed. Blood pressure drops over a relatively short period of time. Considering the risk to health of being very overweight, they are a reasonable alternative.

The problems with all preemptive actions are these:

Someone unwilling to change can defeat any preemptive action. It Is possible, if one is determined, to smoke in the shower, to buy things without a credit card, and to wriggle out of the ropes tying him to the ship's mast. Some patients defeat gastric bypass by eating, painfully, perhaps, enough to stretch their remaining pocket of stomach so that it is big enough for them to gain weight again. Some preemptive actions are easier to defeat than others, but all can be defeated.

It is hard, for the reasons mentioned above, to get anyone to try these strategies in the first place. That person really has to want to change and, also, has to be optimistic enough, and realistic enough, to give these new ways of behaving a try. I will say something later on about motivating patients; but the fact is, for the most part, a successful dieter is somebody who has already found his/her own reasons for being motivated.

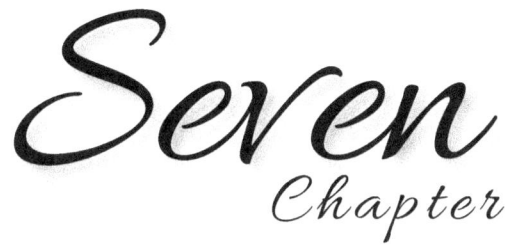

Seven
Chapter

STUFFING YOURSELF.

 he secret for dieting successfully— which means reaching and staying   at your proper weight— is to eat whenever you feel hungry, BUT TO EAT ONLY FOODS THAT WILL NOT MAKE YOU FAT. During the initial stage of the diet, when you are trying to lose weight, you will have to STUFF YOURSELF WITH THESE FOODS in order to stop yourself from eating all those foods you usually eat and that have caused you to become overweight. Stuffing yourself is a preemptive action. Among those foods best suited for this purpose are soups, salads, and cereals. Please note that these are ordinary foods which eaten in ordinary ways do nothing to stop overeating. Indeed, salads are usually served in restaurants as a beginning to a meal which might then include a large meat entrée, bread and butter, wine and desert. Obviously, eating a salad in the portions usually served in a restaurant will do nothing to deter further eating. When I say that you have to stuff yourself with salads, I mean that you have to eat them until you have the feeling you *cannot* eat any more. The amount of salad that might represent is probably, for most people, four to five times what would be served in a restaurant. I understand that you don't *feel like* eating that much salad. You would prefer the steak that appears later on in the menu or that everyone else is eating at the barbecue. But you can do it. Experience has demonstrated to me over and over again that it is easier for someone to stuff himself/herself with food than simply to try to eat high-caloric foods in smaller amounts. You have probably learned by your own experience that eating less of something is hard to do, and for most people impossible to do indefinitely.

But eating salads does not have to be an unpleasant chore. Feeling stuffed in inherently unpleasant, but not so unpleasant that people don't do it regularly at Thanksgiving and on other occasions. Later on, during the time you are trying only to maintain your proper weight, you will not have to eat anything to the point of feeling stuffed. But by that time, if you take care to prepare your salads carefully, you will have come to like salads! Just as learning to like exercise may take two to three months of exercising, coming to prefer salads to steak may very well take somewhat more than six months; but that unbelievable transition will take place. If you stay on the diet long enough to find this out for yourself.

MEASURING PROGRESS

The goal of proper dieting is not to lose weight, and certainly not to lose it as fast as possible; it is to get to a proper weight in a way that allows for new habits of eating to be established. The goal is to be slender, comfortably, forever. So, measuring progress by what the scale says day to day misses the point. Weight varies from day to day for all kinds of reasons. The way to measure progress is: did I eat properly today? And did I exercise properly today? The dieter should feel good if he/she has dieted properly for a week *even if the scale suggests that no weight has been lost.* To an extent, fat may have been lost and replaced by muscle, which weighs more. However, if no weight has been lost over a two to three week period, it is plain that that person, for any of a number of possible reasons, is eating too much or not exercising enough. Some people have to eat less than others to lose weight, or exercise more. A reasonable way of keeping track of all this is to weigh yourself once a week. Determining your weight to a fraction of a pound by weighing yourself every day at exactly the right time, before you have eaten, is a waste of time.

SOUPS, SALADS, AND CEREALS

There are particular advantages to soups, salads, and cereals, although other low density foods can also be used to stuff yourself. Soups are interesting. The solid ingredients in a soup and the fluids that they are cooked with ingested separately seem to cause more weight gain (and are less suitable for dieting) than when they are made into a soup. The reason probably is that stomach emptying time is delayed by drinking a soup. Drinking water before meals, as some people do, to diminish their appetite does not work as well since water is absorbed directly through the stomach. There are very good low-calorie soups. Making an entire meal out of soup does not represent a sacrifice.

Salads are at the heart of any diet. During the active phase of losing weight these salads should not have meats incorporated in them. Salads can nevertheless be tasty and varied, depending on the dressings. A great variety of greens and fruits can be used. Once the transition is made to a maintenance diet, all sorts of meats, fish, nuts and practically anything, can be used to flavor the salads without their having anywhere near the number of calories that would once again encourage weight gain.

Once someone is willing to give them a try, cereals can be found to be a good snack. Some cereals, like granola, have more calories than brans; but even granola is satisfactory since it is so filling. Some successful dieters eat cereals before lunch, in the middle of the day and, sometimes, in the middle of the night. Of course, these should have no extra sugar added. I think it is sensible to make them as varied as possible, with skimmed milk and any sort of fruit or berries. Bananas are okay. I like blueberries or peaches. Cereals should be continued into the maintenance diet.

Eating these foods can be a pleasurable experience. If these are not your favorite foods, (and if you are fat, they are not) keep in mind that food tastes change. Give yourself a chance to like them.

A Brief History of Vegetables by Warren Goodman

The history of civilization is arguably the history of food, especially vegetables. Potatoes and corn, for example, allowed the population growth essential to the rise of different cultures. When crops failed, often the societies based on the cultivation of those foods also failed.

In the beginning, man was primarily a hunter-gatherer, which meant that human beings lived by hunting, scavenging, and gathering nuts, berries and other low-lying vegetables. These foods were eaten after being processed by cutting and cooking. Cooking was so central to the evolution of man that he is often described as "the cooking ape." The cultivation of vegetables that were discovered to be nutritious led to human beings settling down in one area or another, and eventually to the development of advanced cultures. While food in any form was valued, vegetables in the form of crops were critical to mankind's development. We are all the inheritors of that knowledge.

Edible plants can be divided as follows:

From the sea: Primarily seaweed (algae), now known in their politically correct form, "sea vegetables."

From the land: Classic vegetables including potatoes and their kin, eggplants, peppers and tomatoes, squash, cruciferous vegetables (broccoli, cauliflower, kale) nuts and seeds, peas and beans, herbs, beets, spinach and its relatives, grains(corn, rice, wheat, barley), mushrooms (technically not plants since they lack chlorophyll, the green pigment), stems (e.g., celery), roots and other tubers (e.g., celery root, carrots, parsnips, sweet potatoes and jicama) and, of course, man-made products derived from vegetable sources, such as tofu and scitan.

Fruits, a specific part of a vegetable, are delicious and nutritious, but are generally not as chock- full of nutrients as the other vegetables mentioned above. That being said, there are some rather non-nutritious but bulky vegetables, such as iceberg lettuce and celery, which are mostly water and are filling. They can be made more caloric, unfortunately, by slathering on gooey, fatty dressings, such as mayonnaise-based sauces or other oils.

Vegetables in their unadulterated form are delicious and nutritious. Usually they are low in fat. Exceptions include avocado, olives, nuts and soybeans. These are relatively high in fat. Therefore, they work well as supplements but not as the staples of a balanced diet. Other energy-dense foods include corn, oats and wheat. Even in whole, unpulverized and unbleached form, they are relatively high-caloric and might best be eaten in moderation and balanced in conjunction with less energy dense, classic, green vegetables. At the heart of the Stuff Yourself Diet are the green, and sometimes, red, yellow, and orange, vegetables.

SOUPS, SALADS AND CEREALS.

SOUPS:

I like using a pressure cooker for soups and stews. This method is almost exactly opposite to the more familiar slow cooker, the "Crock Pot." Soups and stews cook in minutes instead of hours. Even without a pressure cooker, though, the soups mentioned below cook with traditional methods in a relatively short period of time.

Recent research has shown that adding pureed vegetable to soups and stews makes them subjectively more filling.

Roasted Chicken Broth: Buy a pre-cooked roasted chicken. Take all the meat off it. Throw the bones, skin, and the juices in the container into a pot and cover with water. Boil for 10 minutes. Let cool. Drain in a colander and throw away everything but the broth. It will have a deep, versatile, roasted flavor and will congeal like Jello when refrigerated because it is rich with collagen which will melt when cooked. Keeps in refrigerator for two weeks.

Avogolemono: A Greek classic that is great with, or without, rice, pasta, extra vegetables, pureed vegetables, beans, etc. Simply simmer chicken broth with lemon juice, sugar and salt to taste, and a beaten egg (one egg per serving.) Toss in a bit of pre-cooked chicken. Could easily be made with vegetable broth instead of chicken broth.

"Mother Goodman's Chicken Soup": Get a pre-cooked roasted chicken. Hot, cold, it doesn't matter.

1. Take as much meat off the bird as possible and reserve separately.

2. Put carcass, bones, skin, fat, and the juices from the container into a pot and fill with water to within an inch of the top of the pot.

3. Bring to a boil for 10 minutes.

4. Strain into a clean container by pouring through a colander. This roasted chicken broth will taste different than ordinary chicken broth from raw chicken. It is a versatile ingredient which keeps for two weeks in the refrigerator and can serve as the basis for soup, deglazing a cooking pan, or as an instant flavor booster to cooked vegetables, grains, pasta or stews.

5. Convert into Mother Goodman's chicken soup by cooking onions, carrots, parsley or dill, lima beans, parsnips or almost anything else, salting to taste, and adding some of the reserved pre-roasted chicken.

Quick chicken/vegetable soup: Start with any broth, add some Parmesan or Romano cheese (grated, chunk, or even the rind alone, which I prefer.) Add pre-cooked carrots, peppers and/or a handful of precooked soybeans, accompanied, if you wish, with some garlic or other spice/herb you may have on hand. Don't use a lot. Simmer for 10 minutes.

Lablani (Tunisian Chicken Soup): This is much simpler than it sounds. Bring chicken broth to a boil with a few squirts of lemon juice, a small handful of chopped onions and a few pinches of dry or fresh parsley. Salt to taste. Add two pinches of sage or bay leaf. Add one can of drained, canned chickpeas. Simmer for 5 or 10 minutes with an egg cracked carefully into the broth. Ideally, the egg should be cooked so that the yolk is slightly more than soft-boiled, and still runny. Serve with some capers and hot sauce to taste. The vinegar from the capers cuts the richness of the soup. The egg can be omitted, or used to a lesser or greater amount, as you like.

Black Bean Soup: Canned, cooked black beans are practically in soup/stew form instantly, right out of the can. Simmer with a little broth of almost any type (vegetarian, chicken, pork or beef.) Add a little bay leaf (use ground bay leaf or remove the whole leaf after cooking) or sage. You can add a vegetarian sausage and a little chopped onion for a satisfying main course or side dish.

Miso: Simmer a few pieces of kelp (kombu, in the Asian market) until brothy, maybe 5 minutes. Discard kelp. Add a spoon or two of miso paste and dissolve in broth. Simmer. Add a bit of chopped firm or extra-firm tofu, perhaps a bit of spinach or wakanebe seaweed (green and way more delicate than the kombu.) That's it. Eat immediately. Season with a dash of soy sauce to bring out the meatiness, for lack of a better word, of this vegetarian dish. Note: This is an unamic powerhouse which embodies the essence of that exotic word, which means savoriness. The chemical glutamic acid was isolated from kelp by Japanese scientists one hundred years ago. Totally delicious and no MSG headache.

Butternut squash soup: This is, as the saying goes, dead simple. Butternut squash is a pretty versatile vegetable. You can roast it whole, or chopped, or puree it as a side dish. You can make it into a creamy or chunky soup, or add it to lasagna. As a soup it makes a great comfort food. Depending on your level of ambition, you can cook it alone or in combination with carrots, onions, celery, parsnips or chestnuts. Water or broth is fine for the cooking liquid. Throw in a chunk or, even better, a rind of Parmesan or Romano cheese. Using a little olive soil to sauté it is okay. Use a deep enough pot so that when using your immersion blender, you can puree it to the level you like without splashing it all over. (Note: You can also roast or sauté the squash, which will carmelize it and give it a deeper flavor.) This soup definitely fills you up.

Broccoli soup: Add some pre-cooked broccoli (read: leftover cooked broccoli) into broth, cook until hot, then use immersion blender to puree right in the cooking pot to make a smooth soup. This soup is great with sautéed garlic and Parmesan.

Ham broth: A hambone or ham hock simmered in water gives a ton of flavor. A classic with beans, great with almost any root vegetables or stems (celery, carrots, onion.)

Bean soups, like Lentils and White Beans: Cook a bit slowly; but don't worry about overcooking. They are almost impossible to ruin. You need a combination of fresh and dry ingredients. Apply heat for a few hours and then enjoy. This soup is usually better the next day.

Mirepoix: The "Holy Trinity" of chopped onion, scallion or shallot, or, if you like, celery and bell pepper (usually green pepper), forms a delicious basis for many dishes, soups and stews.

SALADS

Everyone knows salads are basically cold preparations or combinations of food, usually employing vegetables as a base. I feel it is important not to allow salad dressing to dominate the salad and blast the eater with a heavy hit of oils in the dressing. We are preparing a line of salad dressings under the "Stuff Yourself Diet" label; and these should be available soon.

Basic Salad Dressing Mixture: Here is my nonfat recipe. A teaspoonful of pasteurized (pre-packed) egg whites, vinegar, flavorings like mustard, garlic, salt and pepper. That's it. I tend to dress my salads with vinegar, lemon/lime juice, hot sauce and mustard. I try to avoid oils. Even though they have a great mouthfeel, they are simply too caloric—and I mean intensely caloric. Nonfat mayonnaise works also.

Mustard and nonfat yogurt or sour cream makes a nice, practically effortless, dressing with a bit of salt and pepper.

High-Protein, low-fat Convenience Foods: These make great additions to soups and salads. The meats should be used in small amounts, mostly as flavorings and primarily in a maintenance diet. For stuffing yourself, try to stick mainly to vegetables. Raw vegetables work best.

Foods that can be added to salads.

Grilled, steamed, boiled or roast chicken.

- Cooked soybeans (edamame).
- Canned soybeans or chickpeas; nuts.
- Roasted or boiled corn
- Chapped hard cheese (in moderation, e.g., Parmesan, Romano, Swiss)
- Hard-cooked eggs.
- Roast pork.
- Lean steak or roast beef.
- Smoked or roasted turkey
- Smoked salmon.
- Anchovies (drained of oil).
- Tuna (similarly drained of oil).

I particularly recommend the following salads which are absurdly easy to prepare:

- Chopped salad: vegetable stems (broccoli, cauliflower, asparagus, celery and some chopped green and red cabbage) are much easier to chew when chopped. They can be the basis for a nice salad dressed with a bit of red wine or balsamic vinegar, with some slightly less chewy ingredients like poultry, cheese and tomatoes. Use plenty of vegetables to get the benefit of the Stuff Yourself Diet.

- Ceviche seafood salad over lettuce: On an ample base of chopped iceberg or romaine lettuce, you can make a five minute ceviche by marinating boneless, lean white fish (fluke, flounder, tilapia, sea bass) in lime juice with some chopped red onion, adding chili peppers, garlic, salt, pepper and chopped fresh cilantro to taste. It works well with raw shrimp or scallops, too. This can be marinated for up to several hours. Marination in the acidic juice basically pickles the fish and "cooks" it without heat, changing the proteins into a denatured form more akin to traditional cooking methods.

- Seafood salad is a pretty standard recipe using cold, marinated, poached or boiled fresh shrimp, scallops, octopus, squid, and whelk (sea snails) and cooked and refrigerated clams and mussels and some chopped raw red onion. Dress with lemon and a vinaigrette or cocktail sauce (two-thirds ketchup, one-third grated horseradish, a splash of Worcestershire sauce to taste).

- Steak salad: great with a mustard dressing and some onions, peppers and/or green beans along with Romaine lettuce and chopped tomatoes. Can easily be turned into a fresh tuna salad using chunk grilled or jarred tuna (drain oil), chicken, or almost any other kind of salad (chicken, bean) as fast as it takes someone to think of what they want for lunch.

- Spinach salad is a classic. However, instead of a fatty bacon dressing, I recommend a mustard-based or curry-based dressing with some citrus, and perhaps a sprinkle of crumbled bacon which has been cooked and defatted. It is sold in little bits, crushed almost to a powder in a small jar or can. Bacon in that form lasts a long time. A little goes a long way as a flavoring. And it is real bacon, rather than an imitation.

- Other vegetables. I like fennel as a great all-around addition to salads. It can also be served as a crudités with with a light yogurt dip.

CEREALS AND GRAINS:

Cereals are somewhat problematic since many people in the United States automatically link "cereal" with breakfast. We must get past that prejudice and open our minds and stomachs to the many ancient and modern grains which are healthful, delicious and nutritious. These include amaranth, quinoa, and barley, to name a few.

- Oatmeal: This is a basic and essential grain. The less pulverized it is, the better. The more pulverized, the faster it will cook, but it becomes gloppy and, I think, unpleasant, more like baby food. Of course, people still love it in instant form, but in its unadulterated form it is more like risotto. I particularly like a parcooked version of the "steel cut" oats which cook in under 10 minutes, as opposed to almost 30 minutes for the basic unadulterated form. While oatmeal is a breakfast classic, it can be used also as a base or pilaf with grilled shrimp and any other animal protein, such as a small, lean salmon filet. Four ounces, grilled, serves nicely. It can be dressed with a light tomato sauce or vinaigrette, and chopped parsley or dill.
- Rice—so many kinds, so little time. Here's a short list: Brown is beautiful, and there are many varieties to choose from, including

Japanese black rice. Of course, the starchy, tender rice used for paella and risotto (Arborio or Carnaroli) is delicious, but rather heavy. Risotto, in particular, is often full of starch, wine, oil, cheese, etc.; so it should be eaten in very small portions. There are many colored varieties of rice which are naturally more flavorful and healthful as they have their bran layer intact, not polished away.

- Wild rice—is a misnomer, as it is not really a rice, but more like a grass. Still, it makes a great side dish, or, if cold, a great salad. It stands up to dried cranberries, slivered almonds, or chopped celery, hot or cold.
- Barley—this makes a great pilaf also, and each grain holds its integrity.
- Quinoa—several varieties of this ancient, high protein Aztec "super-grain" now exist, such as red and black. There is really little difference in flavor between them.
- Amaranth—a versatile grain, easy to find, with a solid nutritional profile.
- Wheatberries—a little hard to find but worth it, with a toothsome, firm texture. They stand up to dressing and don't get soggy.

All grains make a great pilaf or bed for hot or cold vegetables or meats. Chicken broth can be used as a cooking liquid or as an addition. It is flavorful and goes well with a large variety of foods.

FRUITY ADDITIONS TO GRAINS:

Ordinary cereals can be varied by adding any familiar fruit. These include berries of all sorts and citrus wedges. Apples, bananas, pears, apricots and so on are commonly used. In fact, any fruit at all is fine. Middle Eastern recipes include dried raisins, currants, figs and dates. These are usually rehydrated and cooked with the grains. Cereals can be garnished with cold pomegranate seeds or orange slices. Fennel can be chopped and added to a pilaf for a delicious, slightly herbal taste of licorice. Of course, a small amount of chopped or slivered nuts (almonds, walnuts, hazelnuts) will also add some interesting texture and variety. I also like adding chopped vegetables like peppers to grains.

Other foods, including fluids, can be used to stuff yourself; but most of the foods that work best are either soups, salads or cereals. The stuffed feeling lasts longer.

We have already covered the benefits of salads, which in my mind function as a blank slate on which we may combine and recombine textures and flavors, using meat as a condiment, if at all. They can be a main dish or a side dish. They travel well and last quite a while. Just don't make the mistake of dressing a salad and expecting it to stay crisp hours later. We suggest it will still be crisp hours later). Besides salads, chopped bell pepper, onion and celery form a frequent and delicous basis for many soups and stews.

The benefits of soups are similar in that meats can be used in them as condiments or ingredients, which can then be easily defatted by refrigeration of with a few paper towels floated on top of the soup after it comes to rest. The soup then can function as a blank slate in which vegetables (including legumes), meat, or noodles can easily be adjusted to be more or less dominant in the soup. In addition, almost all chunky soups can be converted from soup to stew and back again by the subtraction or addition of water or broth. Soups can be either a main dish or a side dish. We recommend that soups also be subjected to the same "vinegar, mustard and hot sauce" treatment given to salad dressings in order to adjust spiciness and simulate mouthfeel without oil or fattiness. Spicy soups, and spicy stews such as chili, can be rather easily tailored to the desired degree of spiciness by the addition of chili peppers, ground chili, or similar   Sour ingredients like kimchi, pickled capers, and sauerkraut can quickly tweak the soup and turn it into something completely different, with a puckery, vinegary zing that plays off oiliness or sweetness of carmelized vegetables such as onions or turnips. Sauerkraut, preserved cabbage, makes a great dish with some broth, chopped sautéed vegetables, and bits of lean pork, sausage or chicken. A sprinkling of Hungarian Smoked Paprika into the stew (mix in lowfat sour cream or yogurt at end when cooling) makes a great Paprikash.

The benefits of grains are similar in that they can serve as a textural canvas and often have a toothsome nuttiness and chewiness which can either be sweet or savory, hot or cold. Grains, like salads and soups, can also be easily elevated from side dish to main course; and are equally good plain, with few additions, or with major additions of ingredients such as meat, tofu, shrimp, vegetables or noodles. They also can be subjected to the same "vinegar, mustard and hot sauce" treatment to change the essential character and nature of the dish.   For example, parcooked chopped broccoli or kale can be added to a dish of wild rice, wheatberries, or barley, with some chopped grilled sausage, shrimp, or other protein, and perhaps some dried cherries or cranberries, to give a colorful, phytochemical (literally "plant-chemical") powerhouse. Spiced with basic garlic, onion, salt and pepper, this dish can easily be further tweaked with some mushrooms, potatoes, or celery. Mushrooms, particularly shitakes, and a sprinkling of soy sauce can be a great addition to almost any stew, whether wine-fortified, broth-tweaked, tomato-based, or even cream-based (not typically a low-fat option, but still really good with the soy-shitakes.)

More thoughts about dieting: by F. Neuman M.D.

Studies indicate that there is an optimum rate of weight loss. People who lose more than two pounds a week are more likely to gain it back. Attempting to jump-start a diet is a bad idea. Naturally, people would like to start a race with a head start, but it leads to disappointment only a few months down the road since a rapid pace of weight loss cannot, and should not, be maintained. What was said above about exercise applies also to eating a sensible diet. *It takes time for someone's tastes to change.* Therefore, the dieter should approach a maintenance diet slowly. But tastes do change! I don't think it is possible to remain permanently on a diet that is uninteresting and unsatisfying. Most dieters think that if they can only get down to their proper weight, they can then manage their weight by eating less of everything. Their own experience suggests that this will not work. Certainly it is not possible to go through life hungry.

The final diet that someone settles down to should have the following character:

1. No food should be completely excluded. As soon as a food is completely off-limits, it becomes more enticing. High caloric (high density) foods should be used sparingly.

2. The diet should include a lot of fish and only a little meat. There should be a lot of vegetable and fruit dishes. These can be prepared in an astonishingly wide variety of ways.

3. Meals should start with soup. Soup, salads and cereals, which are critical in the early stages of dieting, should be integrated also into a permanent, maintenance diet.

4. The diet should be varied. People have to look forward to eating.

5. Snacks should always be immediately available. Fruit is best. High caloric snacks should not be kept around the house and certainly not "for the sake of the children." If children develop healthy eating habits when young, they won't have to struggle to change those habits later in life.

6. Diet sodas, paradoxically, seem to cause weight gain. Still, I think it is reasonable to drink a big glass of diet soda before going out for dinner. Your mother was right; it ruins your appetite.

7. There has to be some understanding of the fact that *everyone* will go off the diet from time to time. This is not a bad thing to do, and, therefore, it should not lead to anyone binging because he/she has already already eaten "too much" of the wrong food.

8. More specifically, the diet should include some foods that when eaten to excess would be undesirable. A couple of cookies are fine. Eating the whole box of cookies is bad. I think it is possible to learn how to avoid bingeing by literally practicing eating small amounts of cookies or ice cream and then walking away from the table. Knowing that the basic diet has not been violated makes all the difference.

9. The particular diet the dieter settles on can be different from one person to the next. There is room for trying different foods in different amounts. As I said before, dieting is like going downstream in a boat; the traveler can move from one place to another in the boat; he just can't jump over the side.

10. At the end of a meal, no one should be hungry.

The proper *way* to eat

1. People should eat whenever they are hungry, before meals, during meals and at other times. People should *not* eat when they are not hungry, even if they are in the middle of a meal.

2. In general, people should eat frequently, but in small portions. It is better to take another portion, than take too much in the first place.

3. It is a good idea to leave some food uneaten. People inclined to be over-weight have to get out of the habit of eating what is on their plate just because it *is* on the plate. Of course, they should not finish what is uneaten on *other people's* plates.

4. They should eat slowly. It is desirable eventually to eat without paying much attention to the process, but since everyone who is fat tends to eat quickly, it is sensible to make a special effort to eat slowly, for the reasons given previously: it takes a while for the brain to know that the stomach has eaten enough.

5. Eating in our culture (and probably every other culture) is a social occasion. Concentrate on talking to other people. Take every opportunity to interrupt the process of eating. Get up from the table. Make a telephone call. If that seems rude, apologize.

6. A psychological trick that is sometimes suggested is to use smaller plates. Get it? A small plate makes the food look bigger. I think whoever thought of this idea first was probably influenced by Alice in Wonderland. I imagine someone sitting at a small table, eating with small utensils and drinking from a small glass and feeling even more huge than usual. I don't think this works; but you can give it a try.

The Maintenance Diet by Warren Goodman

These are recipes that are interesting, infinitely variable, and appropriate for maintenance on the Stuff Yourself Diet.

SALADS:

People who enjoy fish and shellfish can easily consume these protein sources in many ways. We suggest salads because fish and shellfish cook so rapidly that they are practically convenience foods; indeed, many fish and shellfish are readily available in pre-cooked or ready-to-eat forms. Ready-to-eat is fine. The purpose of this book of this book is not to argue in favor of one kind of food or another, fresh or ready to eat. Organic or not. That being said, you can source your own food, and combine it however you like; we simply offer a plan and some recipes which can naturally be modified or substituted:

Grilled fish or shellfish (hot) over cold salad;

Cold fish or shellfish cold salad.

Grillled fish can be in steak, filet or whole fish form. We suggest salmon, swordfish, mahi-mahi, halibut, striped bass, bluefish or Chilean sea bass. If using delicate filets of a flatfish like flounder or sole, you might prefer to grill it in foil. If using fresh herbs like parsley, basil and cilantro, with or without lemon or lime slices, the fish can be wrapped in a foil packet with the fruit and vegetables and grilled together in a unit; or the filet can be simply rolled around the vegetables. Or the body cavity of a whole fish can be stuffed with sliced lemon, lime and herbs, and drizzled with a a little olive oil. Shellfish, shrimp, scallops or squid are lean, can be marinaded or not, and cook very rapidly and with a little char to them. (N.B.,lobster tends to get tough on the grill). Sometimes all that is needed is a squeeze of lemon juice, or a light sprinkle of soy sauce. Similarly, hot sauce, garlic salt or garlic powder, or a tiny bit of oil, will get the sear working. HINT: make sure the grill is clean (scraped when hot and lightly oiled by wiping oil on with a paper towel) and very, very hot before cooking. The food will then cook very rapidly. Remember to clean the grill next time too.

Alternatively: grill chicken or turkey, or use smoked salmon, smoked bluefish, smoked trout, or smoked shrimp.

For the salad base: we suggest using a bed of lettuce, bell peppers, spinach, and chopped vegetables (including broccoli and cauliflower, especially the stems.) Steam, par-cook or microwave for a minute or two to make them firmer and more toothsome. Use zucchini, cucumber, tomato, and carrot, or mixed chopped/torn green herbs as a bed, which can include parsley, fennel, scallion, cilantro and basil. Lightly sauteed spinach, chard, or kale work well too and require minimum oil. They can be cooked in this manner with a splash of broth, water, wine, or vinegar.

Be sure to add to the salad some fruit (fresh, such as grapes or berries; or dried, such as raisins, dried cranberries, chopped dried pears, or chopped dried tomatoes,) You can add cheese, if you like, grated or shredded, either neutral, light, or heavier in flavor, and/or a sprinkle of nuts (pignoli, walnut, almonds). You can add chopped or torn-up green herbs to the salad.

SAUCES:

Fish and shellfish marry well with citrus fruits like lemon and lime. Less traditionally, orange and grapefruit can also be incorporated into fish dishes. It is worth noting, that grapefruit is sometimes contraindicated for people taking certain medications. Beyond that, and in general, you should check your medicines with your doctor or pharmacist for any dietary limitations or restrictions.

Sauces:

We suggest the following low-fat sauces which are still creamy but also somewhat tart:

a. Yogurt-based sauce: use non-fat or low-fat yogurt or sour cream, to which you can mix chopped herbs (basil—as in a low-fat pesto; and/or scallion, cilantro, and jalapeno pepper.) You can add some lemon, salt, pepper and a little sugar too. Other yogurt-based sauces incorporate mustard, which is perfectly soluble in all proportions. Any type of hot sauce can be mixed in. Curry, mentioned previously, also makes a great instant sauce when mixed with low-fat mayonnaise or yogurt. Hot sauce also mixes perfectly with yogurt. Experiment to find the best combination that works for you.

b. Greens-based sauces—as mentioned above, a type of salsa verde. A combination of fresh greens, some jalapeno, green pepper, and a bit of oil or nonfat yogurt. Add some acid like vinegar or lemon juice (1 tablespoon) and also a splash or two of pasteurized egg whites. This will work well blended together and is also colorful. For a crazy-easy, green-based sauce, we suggest this variation of the ginger-scallion sauce developed by NY Noodletown and David Chang in New York City. It is more like a pesto, but needs little oil and packs a lot of flavor. So, get a jar of pickled, sliced sushi-type ginger (pink or white, it doesn't matter) and puree one or two ounces of it with an immersion blender or regular blender. Use the juice. Add some neutral oil like grapeseed or vegetable oil, so that the flavor of the oil doesn't fight the pesto. Get a bunch or two of scallions and trim off the root ends. Blend and add some vinegar (any type, really, but recipes tend to call for less-strongly flavored vinegars such as sherry or rice vinegar), a splash of soy sauce and oil; and you may also use pasteurized egg whites as a source of liquid to enhance the blending. Add salt, pepper, and sugar to taste.

c. "Vinaigrette" based: not a true vinaigrette since there is no oil needed. Use pasteurized egg white, mustard and vinegar, salt and pepper. We repeat: no oil is necessary. We recommend using a splash or two of egg white, a 1/4-teaspoon of mustard, a half-teaspoon of any vinegar; then add some sliced garlic, chopped onion, scallion or shallot, if you like. Hot sauce is optional. If you want to use Asian-style fish sauce or miso paste, then by all means feel free to do so and take the "vinaigrette" in that direction.

Salads, like most foods, benefit from an interplay of flavors and textures which make the dish more enjoyable and intriguing. For that reason, we suggest using blueberries or strawberries, which often have tart, acid components. Grapes are similar but usually sweet. Grapefruit is also refreshingly tart. We like to use these sweet-acid foods in salads for several reasons:

a. They are low-calorie.

b. They appeal to the palate with varied tastes, textures, and interplay of flavor. They work well with cold vegetables.

c. They pick up sugar or sweetness in dressing or in other ingredients (e.g., beets, nuts) and complement savory components and ingredients.

SOUPS AND STEWS; WHOLE GRAINS AND LEGUMES—DECONSTRUCTED

The principle difference between a soup and a stew is the amount of moisture it contains. Ingredients in a cooked soup often absorb the liquid, making it more like a stew over time. This equilibrium can be changed simply by adding or subtracting water or broth to the thickened soup or stew. Also, soups sometimes have pureed vegetables, making the soup more filling. Whole grains are also good additions to soups and stews. Legumes are, of course, a natural addition. We have made, for example, a grilled chicken and cauliflower stew, Moroccan style. Put 2 lbs. of grilled, sliced chicken into a pan deglazed with 2 tablespoons of red wine vinegar. Add one cauliflower sliced 1/2 inch thick, and parcooked. Add 28 oz. of canned pureed tomatoes, plus a half-teaspoon each of ground sage and ground cinnamon. This dish easily accepts beans, rice, oatmeal, or barley, alone or in combination. The next day just add some water or broth to turn the stew back into soup.

Tofu and the other processed vegan proteins such as seitan, tempeh and textured vegetable protein are useful for people who want to avoid meat for any reason. New advances in food technology are bringing a dramatically improved vegetarian "chicken" closer to the market. Accordingly, these vegetarian processed proteins are excellent ingredients for soups, stews, and in combination with legumes and whole grains.

Beans and other legumes are nutritional phytochemical (plant-chemical) powerhouses and also packed with fiber. Fiber is also an important benefit of whole grain cereals. Fiber is undigestible plant matter and is important especially because many Americans eat far less than the suggested daily amounts of 25 grams for women and 38 grams for men. Fiber is an under-appreciated component of diets. In addition to its health benefits, such as warding off colon cancer. It also seems to have an important calorie-sparing effect that should make fiber a central consideration in any diet.

Schedule "taco night" meals where everyone can assemble their own taco from several ingredients on the table. The prep work is about the same. For this reason, we like making "deconstructed" dinners such as deconstructed chili, deconstructed tacos, and deconstructed paella. They have the benefit of reheating well in whole or in part, and can be combined or recombined into endlessly interesting meals.

Deconstructed Chili: This is a classic American stew of tomatoes, beans and other vegetables, plus ground or chopped beef or other animal protein and spices. Chile can be made from venison, buffalo, turkey, etc.; but there is no reason why it could not be made with processed vegetable protein instead, or even fish or shellfish. These are lean proteins which can easily stand up to strong, hearty spices and flavors. Therefore, we suggest cooking separately first the main protein, then beans/lentils and then a whole grain like barley, brown rice, or wild rice either by steaming, grilling or boiling. If steaming or boiling any ingredient, consider using a chicken or vegetarian broth. Then, one ingredient can be made with a tomato base or stewed tomato sauce, and one ingredient can be spiced. Or the spices can be added to each portion. Some low-fat cheese and non-fat sour cream round out the chili.

Deconstructed Paella: This rice stew of shellfish, poultry, sausage, and vegetables can include quick-grilled garlicky shrimp, or grilled chicken, or low-fat turkey sausage. Stewed peppers with tomato, onion, celery and garlic can be used as a base with barley or some other whole grain or rice. Everyone can make his/her own dish. Have plenty of shrimp on hand, as it is usually a crowd-pleaser.

A final word: by Fredric Neuman, M.D,

I am the Director of the Anxiety and Phobia Center at White Plains Hospital. I have spent most of my professional life dealing with panic attacks and phobias. In fact, I used to be phobic myself. So, what I say about phobias is credible to patients. The nice thing about being phobic, I tell my patients, is that the condition evaporates if they do the right thing. That is certainly not true for depression or schizophrenia or most other psychiatric illnesses. But if someone is afraid of bridges, for example, and is willing to spend enough time on bridges, that fear will surely go away. It doesn't matter whether that person has the right attitude, or the wrong attitude, or has some outlandish idea about bridges being made out of putty. Enough time spent on bridges leads inevitably to being comfortable on a bridge.

Most bridge phobics can be motivated sooner or later to walk and drive across bridges repeatedly, long enough to lose their fear. But it is not an easy process. Even with the encouragement of a credible person, and the example of others who have overcome similar problems, it is difficult for someone accustomed to feel and think a certain way to behave in a new, almost opposite, way. So it is with the Stuff Yourself Diet. Eat too much purposely? Whoever heard of such a thing? This diet works, but only if you really give it a try. For a long enough period of time.

There is, perhaps, one final reason for dieting successfully and maintaining a proper weight from then on: it is really hard to do. Giving up cigarettes is much easier. It is difficult for an alcoholic to give up alcohol, but I think not as difficult as dieting properly. It is possible to avoid alcohol; it is not possible to avoid food. I tell my patients that overcoming my phobias did more for my self-confidence than anything else I ever did; and I think the same applies to successful dieters. The victories we have over ourselves can never be taken away. The ability to struggle on in the face of disappointment or failure makes for character; and ultimately that makes all the difference between success and failure in life.